Innov8

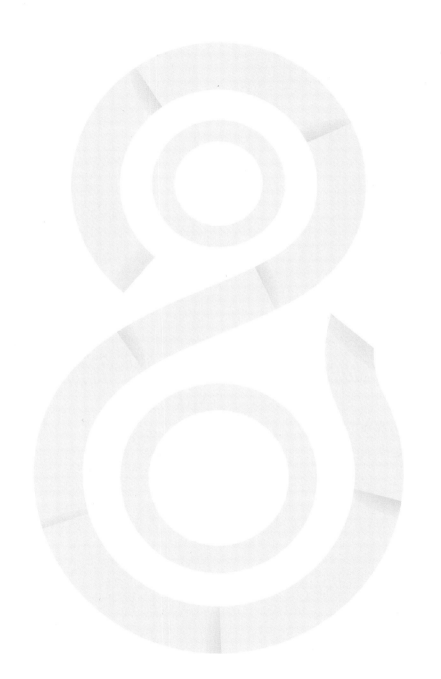

The Innov8 approach for reviewing national health programmes to
leave no one behind

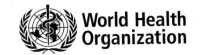

World Health
Organization

Living document, version 2016

WHO Library Cataloguing-in-Publication Data:

Innov8 approach for reviewing national health programmes to leave no one behind: technical handbook.

1.National Health Programs. 2.Health Priorities. 3.Health Equity. 4.Socioeconomic Factors. 5.Gender Identity. 6. Right to Health. 7.Handbooks. I.World Health Organization.

ISBN 978 92 4 151139 1   (NLM classification: WA 540)

Printed in Italy.

Editor: Vivien Stone.

Design and layout: www.paprika-annecy.com

Table of contents

Abbreviations and acronyms

AAAQ	availability, accessibility, acceptability and quality
AFS	adolescent friendly services
ASRH	adolescent sexual and reproductive health
BCC	behavioural change communication
CEDAW	Convention on the Elimination of All Forms of Discrimination against Women
CESCR	Committee on Economic, Social and Cultural Rights
CHD	coronary heart disease
CRC	United Nations Convention on the Rights of the Child
CRPD	United Nations Convention on the Rights of Persons with Disabilities
CSDH	Commission on Social Determinants of Health
FOBT	faecal occult blood testing
GAQ	Gender Analysis Questions
GRAS	Gender Responsive Assessment Scale
HERD	Health Research and Social Development Forum
HFOMC	health facility operation and management committee (Nepal)
HiAP	Health in All Policies

HIV/AIDS	human immunodeficiency virus infection / acquired immune deficiency syndrome
HRBA	human-rights based approach
ICESCR	International Covenant on the Economic, Social and Cultural Rights
IEC	information, education and communication
KISS	keep it simple and sensitive
M&E	monitoring and evaluation
NGO	nongovernmental organization
NORAD	Norwegian Agency for Development Cooperation
RR	relative ratio
SDGs	Sustainable Development Goals
STIs	sexually transmitted diseases
UHC	universal health coverage
UN	United Nations
UN Common Understanding	UN Statement of Common Understanding on Human Rights-Based Approaches to Development Cooperation and Programming
WHO	World Health Organization
WHO/EURO	World Health Organization Regional Office for Europe

Foreword

I recall going on school outings as a child when our teacher would check we were all on the bus by carefully counting heads before we set off. Surprisingly, this early memory of making sure no one was left behind seems relevant now to the infinitely more complex world of global health and development.

"Leave no one behind" is a core principle of the Sustainable Development Goals (SDGs). Equity, human rights and gender equality are central to all the goals, while SDG 3 calls for universal health coverage and health and well-being for all at all ages. To realize this inclusive vision, we have to ensure that everyone makes it on to the bus of the SDGs – by using new approaches and tools that help us identify, and then address, health inequity.

Of course, this is not as straightforward as doing a head count (although counting – through surveys, civil registration and other means – is part of the process). We know that we must strengthen health systems and increase collaboration with non-health sectors. But still more is required. Achieving equitable health coverage, everywhere, requires a transformative approach to the complex and varied challenges that prevent millions from realizing their human right to the highest attainable standard of health – as enshrined in the WHO Constitution of 1948.

Within this context, I welcome the timely publication of this Technical Handbook on the Innov8 approach to reviewing national health programmes to leave no one behind. The Innov8 approach supports the objectives and spirit of the SDGs by helping health professionals to identify health inequities in different country contexts, and to correct them by recalibrating health programmes and interventions.

The eight-step Innov8 review is undertaken in each country by a multidisciplinary national team. It identifies who is being missed by health programmes, the barriers they face and the reasons those barriers exist – including the social determinants of health. It recommends the monitoring activity, partnerships and coordinated intersectoral action needed to ensure that health programmes reach everyone, especially those who have been missed and overlooked in the past. Adaptable to the varied needs of different countries and programmes, Innov8 complements other WHO and UN tools and resources and will help Member States meet their commitments under the SDGs, ensuring that no one is left behind.

The SDGs are an historic opportunity to achieve universal health coverage and genuine equity in access to health services. However, history has taught us that our commitments must be backed by sustained and coherent action across the health sector, and must engage fully with other relevant sectors. WHO is committed to working with countries on these actions to achieve better health for everyone.

Dr Flavia Bustreo
Assistant Director-General
Family, Women's and Children's Health
World Health Organization

Acknowledgements

This handbook is a "living document", encapsulating an approach which has been evolving over a number of years. Building on the stepwise review process' previous iterations by Member States (see below) and the WHO Regional Office for Europe, this evolving iteration of Innov8 was developed under the overarching leadership of Veronica Magar (Team Leader for Gender, Equity, and Human Rights (GER)) and Eugenio Villar (Coordinator for Social Determinants of Health (SDH)). Appreciation goes to Flavia Bustreo (Assistant Director General, Family, Women's, and Children's Health, WHO/HQ) for her strategic direction. Thanks goes to Maria Neira (Director, Public Health, Environmental and Social Determinants of Health) for her inputs.

The conceptualization and technical oversight of a WHO/HQ Innov8 workstream, the commissioning of this handbook to Chilean consultants (Orielle Solar and Patricia Frenz – see next paragraph), the co-authoring of text, the spearheading of the Innov8 piloting and scaling up approach, the oversight of the handbook production and the coordination of the related global meetings was led by Theadora Koller (Technical Officer for Equity on the Gender, Equity and Human Rights team) and Victoria Saint (Technical Officer on the Social Determinants of Health team until July 2015, afterwards as SDH consultant responsible for Innov8).

This Technical Handbook draws substantially from materials conceptualized and pioneered by the Government of Chile during 2008-2010, as part of Chile's national strategy for health equity, to review health programmes to better address health inequities. The Chilean consultants, Orielle Solar and Patricia Frenz, who led work for conceptualization and authorship of the approach in Chile, were commissioned by WHO to further develop the stepwise review process into Innov8, as well as to be advisors and co-facilitators in the pilots of this latest Innov8 iteration. Special acknowledgement also goes to Jeanette Vega, Sanjeev Sridharan and to all Chilean review team members for their contributions to the original stepwise review methodology, upon which Innov8 is based. Thanks is also extended to Jaime Neira for his ideas for an earlier iteration of Innov8.

Innov8 also draws from the experiences of the Ministry of Health, Social Services and Equality of Spain, which conducted a training process with the review of programmes at national and subnational levels in 2010 and 2011, based on the Chilean experience, and developed a Methodological Guide based on this training process. The Spanish Government also partnered with WHO for adaptation of the stepwise review methodology for equity to use in WHO Europe regional activities during 2012-2015, involving in the first application Bulgaria, Montenegro, Serbia and the former Yugoslav Republic of Macedonia and in the second application Albania, Kosovo (in accordance with Security Council resolution 1244, 1999), Romania, Slovakia and Ukraine.

Directly contributing to this version of Innov8, the Spanish Government also co-hosted with WHO/HQ and the WHO Collaborating Centre for Social Inclusion and Health (University of Alicante) the meeting "Methodology for reorienting national health programmes to better address equity, social determinants, gender and human rights" in Alicante, Spain, in July 2014. WHO's gratitude goes to Begoña Merino Merino, Pilar Campos, Ana Gil Luciano, Maria Santaolaya, as well as Daniel La Parra for their strong partnership.

The pilots of the latest iteration of Innov8 during 2014-2015 were executed under the leadership of government-nominated counterparts and WHO Regional and Country/Territory Offices. Special thanks goes to Gita Maya Koemarasakti and Khanchit Limpakarnjanarat, Long Chhun, Rustini Floranita, Prakin Suchaxaya and Benedicte Briot (Indonesia); Pushpa Chaudhary, Ram Padarath Bichha, Ghan Shyam Pokhrel and Jos Vandelaer, Zainab Naimy, Meera Upadhyay, Neena Raina, Prakin Suchaxaya and Benedicte Briot (Nepal); Mohcine Hillali, Fatima-Zahra Mouzouni, Tarik El Ghandour and Yves Souteryand, Samira Jabal and Hala Abou-Taleb (Morocco); and Pilar Campos, Piroska Ostlin and Arta Kuli for coordinating the European training and review processes.

Acknowledgement goes to the following past or present GER/HQ and SDH/HQ staff who provided considerable inputs (by alphabetical order): Gemma Hunting, Aleksandra Kuzmanovic, Nathalie Roebbel, Rebekah Thomas, Nicole Valentine and Joanna Vogel. In addition to the WHO Regional Office staff mentioned in the paragraph above who led the eight pilot applications, the WHO Regional Focal Points for gender, equity, human rights, social determinants of health and vulnerability and health attended the Alicante meeting in 2014 to input to the development of Innov8 and attended the Innov8 Training and Orientation Meeting, in April 2016, Manila, or otherwise engaged in discussions that served to map out application/adaptation options for regional scale up. Many gave valuable suggestions to shape the manual contents and the Innov8 workstream. Particular gratitude goes to the following WHO Regional Office colleagues (in alphabetical order): Hala Abou-Taleb, Britta Baer, Anjana Bhushan, Benedicte Briot, Christine Brown, Anna Coates, Kira Fortune, Suvajee Good, Arta Kuli, Haifa Madi, Oscar Mujica, Davison Munodawafa, Aasa Nihlén, Piroska Ostlin, Hala Sakr, Yvette Seignon-Kandissounon, Prakin Suchaxaya and Isabel Yordi.

This iteration of Innov8 would not have been possible without the substantial financial support received through the NORAD and WHO grant entitled "Operationalizing a Human Rights, Gender and Equity-based Approach to Health Service Delivery", the implementation of which was led by the Gender, Equity and Human Rights team (WHO/HQ) during 2014-2016. Sincere appreciation goes to Bjørg Sandkjaer and Helga Fogstad at NORAD for their strong partnership throughout the process. Other contributions to components of this work are also gratefully acknowledged.

Additional inputs were provided at specific stages of development of the WHO Innov8 workstream, including providing sources to draw from for the handbook or specific pilots, serving as reviewers, giving ideas for gender or human rights integration or drafting specific text, making suggestions for integration in planning cycles and linking to wider health system or programme-specific strengthening initiatives, suggesting synergies with other WHO or UN guidance and resources, or contributing feedback on the design of this handbook as part of a wider Innov8 package and options for its application. Acknowledgement goes to the following additional people for their inputs (in alphabetical order): Valentina Baltag, Anshu Banerjee, Genevieve Begkoyian, Heidi Betts, Carlos Carrera, Venkatraman Chandra-Mouli, Paloma Cuchi, Santiago Esnaola, Isabel Constance Espinosa, David Evans, Anna Gruending, Sofia Gruskin, Ahmad Hosseinpoor, Pojjana Hunchangsith, Kawselyah Juval, Sowmya Kadandale, Rajat Khosla, Usha Kiran Tarigopula, Ines Koffi, Shyama Kuruvilla, Pamela Lupton-Bowers, Uden Maharjan, Bernardo Martorell, Francis McConville, Hernan Julio Montenegro, Rosemary Morgan, Devaki Nambiar, Kumanan Rasanathan, Sundari Ravindran, Gojka Roglic, David Ross, Sherine Shawky, Alaa Shukrallah, Sarah Simpson, Anand Sivasankara Kurup, Allison Smith-Estelle, Marcus Stahlhofer and Astrid Stuckelberger.

WHO is also grateful to the following people, who provided valuable support during their internships to the WHO/HQ Innov8 workstream in the GER and SDH teams: Salma Abdalla, Alexander D'Elia, Sandra Gewalt, Ljiljana Lukic, Lutfi Mohd, Lottie Romero, Sophia Scrimgeour, Veronica Shiroya, Paul Stendahl Dy, Anna Wang and Halit Yapici.

Note on this publication as a "living document"

This handbook is a "living document", and it contains an iteration of Innov8 that has been evolving over a number of years based on country adaptations and applications and a wide range of technical inputs. The Innov8 approach will continue to be refined as the handbook and methodology is adapted and applied in different ways, or certain aspects of it are further developed. Comments on the handbook are welcome and should be sent to innov8@who.int.

Introduction to the Innov8 approach for reviewing health programmes

The Innov8 approach supports the operationalization of the Sustainable Development Goals (SDGs) commitment to leave no one behind and the progressive realization of universal health coverage and the right to health. It does this specifically by identifying ways to take concrete, meaningful and evidence-based programmatic action to address in-country inequities. This technical handbook presents the Innov8 approach, which serves to review how national health programmes can better address equity, gender, human rights and social determinants of health in a way that reflects their overlapping and evolving relation to each other. This type of review is to be aligned with, and feed into, existing national programme planning and review processes. It supports the progressive realization of the right to health by improving programme performance, involving populations affected in decision making and tackling inequities in the achievement of the SDGs.

Ministries of health and others involved in the delivery and design of health programmes in all countries are grappling with the question of how to ensure that no one is left behind. As called for by World Health Assembly resolution 62.14 and the Rio Political Declaration on Social Determinants of Health, many are working to reduce inequities in health service access and health status, including through reforms towards universal health coverage (UHC), enhanced intersectoral action, stronger social participation, and health inequality monitoring. This handbook aims to support these efforts. It responds to the practical question of "how" to move from discussions acknowledging inequities and other shortfalls in the realization of human rights and gender equality, to making actual changes in programmes to tackle those challenges.

The Innov8 approach has the following aims:

- **Enhance capacity through applied learning:** Use health professionals´ ongoing programmatic work to strengthen capacities to understand and apply key concepts and underlying principles to ensure that no one is left behind.

- **Identify entry points for action:** Through a guided analysis conducted by a national review team made up of different stakeholders, identify entry points in a programme so that no one is left behind.

- **Sustained change, improved governance and accountability:** Improve ongoing planning, monitoring, review and evaluation cycles and accountability mechanisms in programmes by integrating measures to leave no one behind.

The handbook's primary target users are national health programme managers and staff at central and subnational levels. The handbook recommends that health programme staff assemble a multidisciplinary review team to conduct the review. This supports participatory approaches as defined in the UN Statement of Common Understanding on Human Rights-Based Approaches to Development Cooperation and Programming (the UN Common Understanding) and WHO's global strategy on people-centered and integrated health services. The review team should include representatives from other relevant parts of the health ministry, research institutes, civil society and nongovernmental organizations (NGOs) and other sectors and stakeholders as appropriate. The review team should also include representatives with expertise in equity, gender, human rights and social determinants of health. Throughout the guide, the potential tasks and activities suggested are directed at this "review team".

The handbook is organized in keeping with the eight steps of the review methodology, which are:

- **Step 1:** Complete the diagnostic checklist;
- **Step 2:** Understand the programme theory;
- **Step 3:** Identify who is being left out by the programme;
- **Step 4:** Identify the barriers and facilitating factors that subpopulations experience;
- **Step 5:** Identify mechanisms generating health inequities;
- **Step 6:** Consider intersectoral action and social participation as central elements;
- **Step 7:** Produce a redesign proposal to act on the review findings; and
- **Step 8:** Strengthen monitoring and evaluation.

The handbook can be used by the review team to guide each step of analysis. The chapters correspond to the steps, and feature descriptions of the step objectives, background reading, activities and examples of the main step outcomes from other programmes that have conducted the review.

The handbook is part of a wider set of resources that contains training facilitator guidance (for capacity-building intervals conducted at key moments during the review), evaluation supports and case studies. This handbook is a "living document", encapsulating an approach which has been evolving over a number of years. It has been developed, tested and adapted by national review teams in different regions of the world to review various types of health programmes (see Box 1). WHO's development of this approach has drawn from country experiences and represents a fluid exchange with national partners for its advancement. Through use in diverse settings, and linked to a community of practice, the Innov8 approach will continue to be refined. Feedback on this handbook as a living document is actively requested by WHO.

The Innov8 review methodology can be adapted and applied in different scenarios. For instance, some options for application and adaptation include:

- Processes for review can be organized by a ministry of health for one or more programmes at national level, and/or be done at subnational level.

- Processes can be facilitated by international agencies through multicountry modalities (where an international organization/partner has a convening role and national review team delegations come from different countries).

- In some contexts, organizers may wish to conduct partial reviews, drawing from only one or more of the steps but not finalizing the full analytical pathway outlined here.

- The Innov8 approach can be extracted and drawn from for incorporation into existing ongoing national reviews of programmes.

- In keeping with the health programme to which it is applied, the approach may be used in conjunction with other WHO normative guidance on that health topic.

Box 1 Evolution of the Innov8 approach

Chile: During 2008–2010, the Ministry of Health of Chile adapted the work of the Priority Public Health Conditions Knowledge Network of WHO's Commission on Social Determinants of Health, combining it with elements of realist evaluation theory. As part of Chile's national strategy for health equity, six health programmes were chosen for reorientation to better address health inequities. The programmes covered cardiovascular health, oral health, workers' health, women's reproductive health, child health and Red Tide. The Chilean Government pioneered the development of the stepwise reorientation approach (five-step reorientation-for-equity approach with selected public health programmes at national and subnational levels). This was done as part of the Chilean Ministry of Health's "13 steps towards equity" strategy.

Spain: In 2010 and 2011, the Ministry of Health, Social Services and Equality of Spain – in conjunction with experts involved in the Chilean process – carried out the training process "Integration of a focus on social determinants of health and health equity into health strategies, programmes and activities at national, regional and local levels". This entailed application and adaptation of the review methodology used in Chile to its national and subnational contexts. This served to review nine national, regional or local health programmes, strategies or sets of activities, including/addressing the national strategic plan for childhood and adolescence; the call for grants on HIV/AIDS prevention and control; the cancer strategy; healthy diet and physical activity programme; health promotion for vulnerable migrants; colorectal screening; youth health; tobacco prevention and control; health education in schools and the Healthy Municipalities Network.

WHO/EURO: In 2012 and 2013, the WHO Regional Office for Europe (EURO) – in collaboration with the Spanish Ministry of Health, Social Services and Equality and the WHO Collaborating Centre for Social Inclusion and Health (University of Alicante) – provided support to the governments of Bulgaria, Montenegro, Serbia, and the former Yugoslav Republic of Macedonia for revision of national strategies and programmes on maternal and child health to better meet the needs and rights of the Roma population (Europe's largest ethnic minority) and other subpopulations experiencing social exclusion. This multicountry process used the Spanish Health Ministry's Methodological Guide to integrate Equity into Health Strategies, Programmes and Activities.

WHO/Headquarters: In 2014–2015, the WHO/HQ units for Gender, Equity, and Human Rights and Social Determinants of Health, in cooperation with persons involved in previous pilots, advanced the stepwise review methodology to further refine it for a range of contexts/scenarios and better incorporate gender and human rights. This led to the development of the Innov8 approach in its current iteration, which underwent further piloting (see below).

Box 1 Evolution of the Innov8 approach (continued)

Indonesia: In 2014 and 2015, the Government of Indonesia co-organized with WHO a process to review how the national neonatal and maternal health action plans could further address equity, gender, human rights and social determinants of health. The findings were integrated into the revised plans and operational approaches. At the time of writing, work is under way to draw from the review methodology for ongoing planning at district level.

WHO/EURO: In 2015, the WHO Regional Office for Europe together with experts from the Spanish Ministry of Health, Social Services and Equality and WHO/HQ, provided support to the governments of Albania, Kosovo (in accordance with Security Council resolution 1244, 1999), Romania, Slovakia and Ukraine for revision of national strategies and programmes on maternal and child health.

Again, the process focused on the Roma population and other subpopulations experiencing social exclusion.

Nepal: In 2015 (with follow up in 2016), the Family Health Division of the Ministry of Health and Population, with support from WHO and partners, applied the review methodology to the national adolescent sexual reproductive health programme. Findings from the review also aimed to feed into the national adolescent health and development strategy.

Morocco: In 2015 (with follow up in 2016), the Government of Morocco, with support from WHO and partners, applied the stepwise review process to the national programme for prevention and control of diabetes, using the Fès Boulmane (now Fès-Meknès) region as a study site.

Innov8 supports health programmes in operationalizing the SDGs' commitment to leave no one behind. Innov8 translates concepts and principles into practical action through a step-by-step approach. It uses frameworks more historically associated with equity through action on the wider social determinants and is informed by human rights principles, health systems strengthening and the gender and health field. Innov8 does not entail an exhaustive nor exclusive analysis using any one of these approaches, which is beyond the scope of this methodology. In its objective to support governments to leave no one behind, Innov8 will continue to evolve as it is adapted to new and changing applications over the coming years. The Innov8 Community of Practice will support learning from and the advancement of the Innov8

approach, and continue to draw from the fields of equity, gender, human rights and social determinants of health, among others.

It should also be emphasized that this Innov8 Handbook complements rather than supercedes other existing tools and processes and capacity building efforts developed by WHO or other partners. While the methodology described here provides a framework to review health programmes, the particular context of a given country and programme will dictate which is the most appropriate tool or approach to apply. In addition, it is important that this WHO resource be considered in conjunction with other health-topic-specific WHO resources for strengthening the programme under review, in keeping with the national planning cycle.

Additional reading and resources

Ministerio de Salud (2010). Documento Técnico I, II, III: Serie de Documentos Técnicos del Rediseño de los Programas desde la Perspectiva de Equidad y Determinantes Sociales. Subsecretaría de Salud Pública: Santiago. [Ministry of Health, Chile (2010). Technical documents I, II and III for supporting the review and redesign of public health programmes from the perspective of equity and social determinants of health. Santiago: Undersecretary for Public Health.] Materials in Spanish only.

Ministry of Health, Social Services and Equality, Spain (2012). Methodological guide to integrate equity into health strategies, programmes and activities. Version 1. Madrid. Available: http://www.msssi.gob.es/profesionales/saludPublica/prevPromocion/promocion/desigualdadSalud/jornadaPresent_Guia2012/docs/Methodological_Guide_Equity_SPAs.pdf (accessed 17 February 2016).

WHO (2013). Integration of social determinants of health and equity into health strategies, programmes and activities: Health equity training process in Spain. Social Determinants of Health discussion paper 9. Geneva: World Health Organization. Available: http://apps.who.int/iris/bitstream/10665/85689/1/9789241505567_eng.pdf (accessed 18 February 2016).

WHO Regional Office for Europe (2014). Review and reorientation of the "Programme for active health protection of mothers and children" for greater health equity in the former Yugoslav Republic of Macedonia. Roma health – case study series no. 2. Copenhagen. Available: http://www.euro.who.int/__data/assets/pdf_file/0008/276479/Review-Programme-active-health-protection-mothers-children-greater-health-equity-en.pdf (accessed 4 March 2016).

WHO Regional Office for Europe (2015). Review and reorientation of the Serbian national programme for early detection of cervical cancer towards greater health equity. Roma health – case study series no. 3. Copenhagen. Available: http://www.euro.who.int/__data/assets/pdf_file/0011/283646/WHO-Roma-Health-Case-Study_low_V7.pdf (accessed 22 February 2016).

Overview of the Innov8 approach

Around the world, national health programmes are striving to ensure that no one is left behind. The Innov8 approach aims to support these efforts. It does so by enabling the generation and application of knowledge, action and mechanisms for a sustained approach towards tackling inequities, promoting the inclusion of gender and advancement of human rights and addressing the social determinants of health.

The Innov8 approach consists of a series of guided activities organized in eight steps. These are shown below.

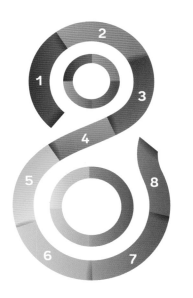

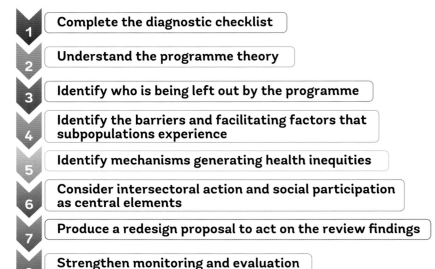

1. **Complete the diagnostic checklist**
2. **Understand the programme theory**
3. **Identify who is being left out by the programme**
4. **Identify the barriers and facilitating factors that subpopulations experience**
5. **Identify mechanisms generating health inequities**
6. **Consider intersectoral action and social participation as central elements**
7. **Produce a redesign proposal to act on the review findings**
8. **Strengthen monitoring and evaluation**

The process begins with Step 1, when the assembled review team produces a diagnostic checklist, which serves as a baseline on which the rest of the analysis is built. In Step 2, the current programme theory about why the programme is expected to produce the desired results is articulated, and then tested in Steps 3 and 4 regarding who is left behind and the presence of barriers, respectively. Step 5 examines the mechanisms generating inequities in the programme, while Step 6 explores how these can be overcome through the enhancement of intersectoral action and social participation. Step 7 focuses on the product of the redesign – programme adjustments and a new programme theory that tackle inequities. These should be gender responsive, address social determinants, and be aligned with human rights principles. Step 8 looks at how to monitor the proposed adjustments to the programme and adjust the ongoing monitoring and evaluation (M&E) framework for sustained attention to leaving no one behind. A more detailed description of Steps 1 to 8 follows.

THE EIGHT STEPS

Step 1 of the 8 steps kickstarts the review process through the completion of a checklist. This checklist summarizes the review team members´ knowledge and experiences and prompts further reflection from equity, gender, rights and social determinants of health perspectives about the programme being reviewed, providing both a baseline of the current situation and inputs for the next steps.

In **Step 2**, the review team analyses the interventions and activities that the programme currently develops and implements. This step focuses on the actual current reality of the programme rather than its aspirations. In Step 2, the review team members elaborate a diagram of the **logic model of the programme**. This sequences and links the activities and who is reached with the programme outputs and short-, medium and long-term outcomes. The logic model diagram helps uncover the **programme theory** – the explanation of how and why the programme is supposed to work and for whom. Understanding how the described activities engage the target population to produce outcomes requires consideration of if and how the programme addresses different operating contexts and the heterogeneous needs of different subpopulations and includes ways to identify and address gender norms, roles and relations. The involvement of those subpopulations furthest behind will be crucial to this exercise, to truly understand the extent to which the programme works for these subpopulations. The current programme theory is tested in the subsequent two steps.

Step 3 centres on who is being left behind by the programme. It aims to identify the subpopulations for whom the programme fails; who are not accessing or fully benefiting from the interventions and activities. It does this through an analysis of available quantitative and qualitative data sources, as well as the team´s own knowledge and experience. As above, this step will benefit from the participation of representatives of target populations who can provide important perspectives of how the programme works in practice and where it needs to be improved. Subpopulations may be characterized by sex, social class, income, education, ethnic minority, migrant status, place of residence (rural/urban), gender identity and sexual orientation, or other relevant characteristics, with due attention to the intersections between these that make some subpopulations at different or more risk of ill health. Step 3 concludes with the identification of one or more specific subpopulations that should be prioritized for the programme review and redesign.

Step 4 examines the reasons why the prioritized subpopulation is not accessing or benefiting, using the lens of the Tanahashi framework for effective coverage (Tanahashi, 1978) to identify barriers – including gender-related barriers – and facilitating factors in the domains of availability, accessibility, acceptability, contact, utilization and effective coverage with quality as a cross-cutting element. These domains relate to select principles of the right to health as defined by the Committee on Economic, Social and Cultural Rights in its General Comment 14 (UN CESCR, 2000).

Step 5 is the most challenging and enriching step of the review process. Prior to Step 5, the review team members systematized available information about the programme, testing whether it works or fails for different subpopulations, considering and addressing gender norms, roles and relations as well as identifying some of the barriers and facilitating factors. This systematized information is further analysed in Step 5 to explain the mechanisms generating inequities, using the WHO framework on social determinants of health (CSDH, 2008). This step also draws on rights analysis of structural causes as well as gender analysis. To do this, the review team members scrutinize how the barriers and facilitating factors are linked to or influenced by social determinants of health including gender (within and beyond the health system). In addition, they examine the causes of the socioeconomic position of the prioritized subpopulation. These analyses examine social stratification mechanisms, linked to the identification of who is left behind (Step 3) and issues of equity of access or discrimination (Step 4). These look at the social, political and economic conditions that result in shortfalls in the creation of an enabling environment for the realization of the right to health. At the end of Step 5, the review team incorporates the information on mechanisms generating inequities and discrimination into their original programme theory to articulate a theory of inequities, which will be redressed in the redesign phase.

Two pillars for tackling health inequities, intersectoral action and social participation, are highlighted in the literature and the WHO framework for action on the social determinants of health (WHO, 2010).

Step 6 examines the way that these critical elements are incorporated in the programme from its planning, implementation, and monitoring and evaluation. The analysis looks at existing mechanisms for participation and the degree to which the target population and the prioritized subpopulation (Step 3) is or is not participating. In addition, the review team considers the influence on access and programme results of other sectors beyond health; specifically, the relationships to relevant social determinants (Step 5), and barriers and facilitating factors (Step 4).

With Step 6, the programme review *per se* concludes and the review team is in a position to identify the entry points and formulate recommendations to redesign the programme. Programme redesign, developed in **Step 7**, commences with identification and prioritization of the changes required to consider the contextual circumstances and differential needs of the prioritized subpopulation, tackling the barriers they face and, most importantly, addressing the mechanisms that explain inequities in programme results. For this, interventions may need to be adjusted, new interventions incorporated (including actions by other sectors), and social participation mechanisms made more robust, with adequate consideration of human rights-based principles. These modifications entail the formulation of **a new programme theory** that improves performance, reduces coverage gaps, compares communities left behind and incorporates other measures to address equity, gender, human rights and social determinants.

Once the proposed changes in the programme are defined, **Step 8** examines relevant M&E issues. One activity in this step looks at the M&E mechanisms that need to be in place to identify whether the proposed adjustments to the programme are reaching the intended aim. Indicators and appropriate sources, both qualitative and quantitative and state and non-state, are essential to support M&E. The feasibility of the indicators requires a review of the available information and the possibility of stratification and, most likely, the introduction of other changes to generate the necessary information (such as expanding sample sizes). Beyond indicators, participatory approaches to monitoring (e.g. involving communities) should also be considered. Another activity calls for suggestions on how the programme's framework and processes for ongoing M&E can better account for equity, gender, human rights and social determinants considerations (not only in relation to the proposed adjustments to the programme, which may have to do with specific interventions for the prioritized subpopulation only). By taking this wider view, the programme's M&E framework and ongoing reviews will have sustained capacity for identification of the subpopulations being missed, the barriers they face, etc. This enables Innov8 to contribute to long-term strengthened capacity for reducing inequities and coverage gaps, responding to the different health needs of women and men, boys and girls and addressing gender norms, roles and relations that are harmful to health, and fulfilling progressive realization of the right to health.

Figure 1 captures the analytical pathway between the steps and also highlights the evolution of the programme's "theory" to be able to tackle inequities.

Figure 1 Analytical pathway through the eight steps of Innov8

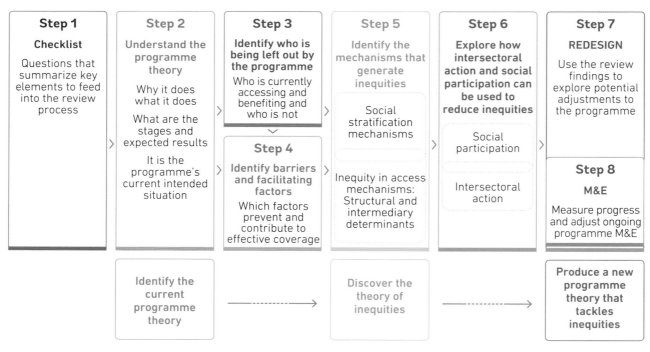

GUIDING PRINCIPLES

The guiding principles of the Innov8 approach are:

• A "learning by doing" approach, usually accompanied by a facilitator team, where the health professionals' knowledge of ongoing programmatic work is the starting point of a transformative process.

• The basis of the review and redesign is a critical analysis of the programme's theory. Programmes are always based on some theory that originates with an understanding of what gives rise to the problem and speculates on how changes may be made to these patterns (Pawson & Tilley, 2004).

• Through the direct experience of developing this critical analysis, using the method's guided activities, current programme theory and practice is challenged in relation to the inclusion of equity, gender, human rights and social determinants, while strengthening participants' capacities for practical application of key related concepts, frameworks and underlying principles.

• The emphasis is on transformative change and developing concrete solutions to programme design and implementation problems, through identification of entry points to ensure that the programme leaves no one behind.

• Sustainability and potential for continuous improvement is achieved by integrating equity, gender, human rights and social determinants of health issues in the programme's ongoing planning, monitoring, review and evaluation cycles.

• Reinforcing a population health perspective to override the prevailing ideological bias towards the individual, based on human rights principles and robust analytical frameworks on the causes of health inequities in general, as well as those associated with gender (Beaglehole & Bonita, 2004).

Innov8 draws from **theory-driven approaches to evaluation**, including critical realism. The focus of this type of evaluation is on developing explanations of the social consequences of actions. Realist evaluation produces a greater understanding of **why, where and for whom health programmes work or fail.** It places emphasis on: (i) identifying the mechanisms that produce observable effects of the programme; and (ii) testing these mechanisms and other context variables that may have impacts on the observed effects (Pawson & Tilley, 2004).

Accordingly, Innov8 strives to disentangle complex issues related to the heterogeneity of subpopulation circumstances and needs, the intricacy of health problems and programme responses, and the multiplicity of contextual influences, including the repercussions of other policies and programmes within and outside the health sector. Innov8 attempts to achieve this through a comprehensive, systematic and sequential process that recognizes the complexities of tackling inequities and the realities of programmatic and policy-making processes. The purpose is to identify and introduce the transformative changes needed to improve the health programme and to make it really work for all subpopulations, especially the most vulnerable and marginalized.

REFERENCES

Beaglehole R, Bonita R (2004). Public Health at the Crossroads: Achievements and Prospects. Cambridge, UK: Cambridge University Press. 2nd edition.

CSDH (2008). Closing the gap in a generation: Health equity through action on the social determinants of health. Final Report of the Commission on Social Determinants of Health. Geneva: World Health Organization. Available: http://whqlibdoc. who.int/publications/2008/9789241563703_eng.pdf (accessed 4 March 2016).

Pawson R, Tilley N (2004). Realist evaluation. London: British Cabinet Office. Available: http://www.communitymatters.com.au/ RE_chapter.pdf (accessed 18 February 2016).

Tanahashi T (1978). Health service coverage and its evaluation. Bulletin of the World Health Organization. 1978;56(2):295–303.

Available: http://www.ncbi.nlm.nih.gov/pubmed/96953 (accessed 22 February 2016).

Solar O, Irwin A (2010). A conceptual framework for action on the social determinants of health. Social Determinants of Health Discussion Paper 2 (Policy and Practice). Geneva: World Health Organization. Available: http://www.who.int/sdhconference/ resources/ConceptualframeworkforactiononSDH_eng.pdf (accessed 26 February 2016).

UN CESCR (Committee on Economic, Social and Cultural Rights) (2000). General Comment No. 14: The Right to the Highest Attainable Standard of Health (Art. 12 of the Covenant), 11 August 2000, E/C.12/2000/4. Available: http://www.refworld. org/docid/4538838d0.html (accessed 4 March 2016).

Introduction to applied concepts, principles and frameworks

OVERVIEW

Innov8 draws from and integrates a set of related concepts and principles from the fields of health equity, gender, human rights and social determinants of health. The concepts and principles are introduced in this chapter, with the aim of enabling the review team to have a common understanding. They will be further expanded upon, examined and operationalized throughout the review process and in the corresponding eight steps.

The application of these concepts and principles is supported by several conceptual and normative frameworks, which "provide a language and frame of reference through which reality can be examined and lead theorists [researchers/evaluators] to ask questions that might not otherwise occur" (Judge et al, 1998:3). These include the WHO framework on social determinants of health and the Tanahashi framework

for effective coverage, WHO's work on gender and health as well as the body of international law of human rights and gender equality, and other WHO strategic frameworks.

The chapter examines gender norms, roles and relations and their impact on health. It also looks at some of the key principles of a human rights-based approach to programming as defined in the UN Common Understanding (United Nations 2003). Theory-driven realist evaluation, on which Innov8 is based, is also described. Linked to the concepts, principles and frameworks, the chapter discusses the role of health programmes in addressing health inequities through closing gaps for effective coverage, as well as intersectoral actions and social participation.

Box 2 Useful definitions

The enjoyment of the highest attainable standard of **health conducive to living a life in dignity is one of the fundamental rights** of every human being without distinction of race, religion, political belief, economic or social condition, including gender. The right to health extends not only to timely and appropriate health care but also to the underlying determinants of health (General Comment 14).

Equity in health means that everyone should have a fair chance to achieve their full health potential and that nobody should be disadvantaged in reaching it. **Health inequities** are avoidable and unjust differences in exposure and vulnerability to health risk factors, health-care outcomes and the social and economic consequences of these outcomes.

The **social determinants of health** are the conditions in which people are born, grow, live, work and age, including the health system. These conditions are, in turn, shaped by the distribution of money, power and resources at global, national and local levels, which are influenced by economic and social policy choices.

The underlying social determinants of health inequities are **structural determinants**, which include socioeconomic and political context, structural mechanisms that generate social stratification in society, and the socioeconomic position of the individual. These structural determinants operate through a set of **intermediary determinants** to shape health outcomes, the main categories being material circumstances, psychosocial circumstances, behavioural and/or biological factors, and the health system itself.

Gender refers to the socially constructed norms, roles and relations of and between women, men, boys and girls. Gender also refers to expressions and identities of women, men, boys, girls and gender-diverse people. Gender is inextricable from other social and structural determinants shaping health and equity and can vary across time and place. **Gender analysis** in health identifies, assesses and informs appropriate responses to different needs and asks critical questions to uncover the root causes of gender-based health inequities.

The goal of the **human rights-based approach to health** is that all health policies, strategies and programmes be designed with the objective of progressively improving the enjoyment of all people to the right to health and other health-related human rights (e.g. safe and potable water, sanitation, food, housing). It focuses attention and provides strategies and solutions to redress inequalities, discriminatory practices and unjust power relations, which are often at the heart of inequitable health outcomes.

Theory-driven evaluation is a contextual or holistic assessment of a programme (based on the programme theory), that provides information on how, why, where and for whom health programmes work or fail.

HEALTH EQUITY, GENDER, HUMAN RIGHTS, SOCIAL DETERMINANTS AND THEORY-DRIVEN EVALUATION, AND THEIR RELEVANCE FOR PUBLIC HEALTH PROGRAMMES

Before beginning to review the health programme, a critical starting point is for review team members to develop a basic common understanding of the concepts and principles, to be further developed across the subsequent steps. The concepts are brought together in the Innov8 approach, which is inspired by theory-driven evaluation to support useful, practical and operational analysis of health programmes for leaving no one behind.

This chapter covers the following key applied concepts, principles and frameworks:

- Equity and the right to health;
- Social determinants of health;
- Gender and health;
- Human rights-based approach;
- Conceptual framework of social determinants of health; and
- Theories of evaluation and equity for health programmes.

Equity and the right to health

The enjoyment of the highest attainable standard of health is one of the fundamental rights of every human being without distinction of race, religion, political belief, economic or social condition [including gender] (WHO, 1946). It is an inclusive right – extending to the underlying determinants of health – whose substantive content has been defined by the Committee on Economic, Social and Cultural Rights, and the realization of which is to be progressively achieved. Within this definition, the concept of "equity in health" represents a central thread that, following its original inclusion in the WHO Constitution in 1946, has continued to be represented in international human rights declarations and national health policies, strategies and plans (WHO Regional Office for Europe, 2006; UN CESCR, 2000). Equity is an important concern for human rights. Its corollary principle of human rights law requires that states take all measures necessary to eliminate discrimination, which has the intention or effect of nullifying or impairing the equal enjoyment or exercise of the right to health (UN CESCR, 2000). Grounds of discrimation include ethnicity, race, colour, sex, language, religion, political or other opinion, national or social origin, property, birth, physical or mental disability, health status (including HIV/AIDS), sexual orientation and civil, political, social or other status.

Equity in health is the absence of avoidable, unfair or remediable differences among groups of people, whether those groups are defined socially, economically, demographically or geographically or by other means of stratification (Solar & Irwin, 2010). "Inequities" in health or health service coverage has a moral and ethical dimension and are distinguishable from "inequalities", which is a term used in health to denote only measurable differences. However, the term inequality is used in legal terminology to describe discriminatory acts or measures that breach the prohibition of discrimination. In health, "inequities" refers to differences in health which are unnecessary and avoidable but, in addition, are also considered unfair and unjust (WHO Regional Office for Europe, 2006; Whitehead, 1991; WHO Regional Office for Europe, 1990). As represented in Box 3, quoting Amartya Sen, health inequities are intrinsically linked to wider issues of fairness and justice in society.

Box 3 Amartya Sen on health equity

"Health equity cannot be concerned only with health, seen in isolation. Rather, it must come to grips with the larger issue of fairness and justice in social arrangements, including economic allocations, paying appropriate attention to the role of health in human life and freedom."

Source: Sen, 2002:659.

"Health equity is most certainly not just about the distribution of *health*, not to mention the even narrower focus on the distribution of *health care*."

Reducing inequities in health is acknowledged as central to strong health systems and universal health coverage, the progressive achievement of the right to health, as well as to sustainable social development more broadly. The mechanisms through which health inequities are produced are very complex and "inescapably multidimensional" (Sen, 2002; CSDH, 2008). This makes action to comprehensively address them through policies and programmes a challenge that requires deliberate multilayered analysis to understand, and innovative intersectoral and participatory solutions to tackle.

Realist evaluation's focus on the capacity of the health programme to address context, and hence address the different needs, circumstances and experiences of subpopulations, is useful to tackle health inequities. In Innov8, the focus is not only on improving the health of the most disadvantaged subpopulations (although a review team may choose to use it this way). Rather, the approach facilitates looking at how different subpopulations across the social gradient may be accessing or benefiting less than others from the

health programme. This enables an approach towards health equity that is in keeping with the ultimate aim initially enshrined in the WHO Constitution.

In this handbook, "equity of access" draws from a broad definition of access that includes the analysis of mechanisms that facilitate or limit access from the supply-side (health system) and the demand-side (individual and communities) because of their influence over individuals' decisions and abilities to interact with the health system. The Tanahashi framework for effective coverage (Tanahashi, 1978) orients this process and allows analysis of the interaction of policies of other sectors with the health system and the programme. It enables the review team to identify how interventions to address social determinants can contribute to increasing equity in access and how to integrate a "Health in All Policies" approach within health system activities (WHO, 2013a). The Tanahashi framework is complemented by human rights law, which also looks to these elements of a right to health as a basis for assessing the realization of right to health and identifying relevant duty-bearers.

Social determinants of health

The "social determinants of health" are defined as **the conditions in which people are born, grow, live, work and age, including the health system** (WHO 2011a). These conditions are, in turn, shaped by the distribution of money, power and resources at global, national and local levels, which are influenced by economic and social policy choices. The conceptual framework of the social determinants of health is introduced later in this section, and is used during the review process to assist analysis.

> "Biological expressions of social inequality refers to how people literally embody and biologically express experiences of economic and social inequality, from *in utero* to death, thereby producing social inequalities in health across a wide spectrum of outcomes."
>
> Krieger, 2001:693.

The underlying social determinants of health inequities are **structural determinants**, which include socioeconomic and political context. These are the base of the mechanisms that generate stratification, social class and gender divisions in society, and the resultant socioeconomic position of individuals. The socioeconomic and political context includes aspects such as the labour market, the educational system, political institutions and redistributive policies as well as cultural and societal values, including those related to gender norms, roles and relations. These underlying social determinants of health inequities operate through a set of **intermediary determinants** of health to shape health outcomes. The main categories of intermediary determinants of health are: material circumstances, psychosocial circumstances, behavioural and/or biological factors, and the health system itself.

The need for action on social determinants of health has been gaining increasing recognition and priority over the last 15 years. The work undertaken during the WHO Commission on Social Determinants of Health (2005–2008) considerably raised the profile and consolidated the current thinking and evidence base on this issue (CSDH, 2008). Since then, there has been increasing global efforts by many actors – in the United Nations, multilateral and governmental agencies, academia, civil society and others – to further develop the evidence, political commitment, experiences and best practices related to this agenda. The Rio Political Declaration on Social Determinants of Health was adopted during the World Conference on Social Determinants of Health in 2011 (WHO, 2011c). World Health Assembly resolutions have called for increased action on social determinants of health, including by reorienting the health sector (WHA, 2009; 2012).

While the term "social determinants of health" may be relatively new, the idea that health and disease is socially produced and linked to development, gender norms, human rights and other societal factors is not. The social production of disease is implicitly or explicitly acknowledged in the WHO 1946 Constitution, the 1948 Universal Declaration of Human Rights, the 1966 International Covenant on Economic, Social and Cultural Rights (which flagged the underlying determinants of health as a key component of the right to health), the Declaration of Alma-Ata on primary health care in 1978 and the Ottawa Charter for Health Promotion in 1986.

Gender and health

Gender is a key determinant of health and strongly influences health outcomes for both girls and boys and women and men across the life course, and thus should be given particular consideration. The term "sex" designates characteristics that are biologically determined, while "gender" refers to **socially defined norms, roles and relations of and between women and men** (WHO, 2011b). Gender also refers to expressions and identities of girls, women, men, boys and gender-diverse people. The concept of gender includes five important elements: relational, hierarchical, historical, contextual and institutional. While most people are born either male or female, they are taught norms and behaviours – including how they should interact with others of the same or opposite sex within households, communities and workplaces. When individuals or groups do not "fit" established gender norms, roles or relations, they often face stigma, discriminatory practices or social exclusion – all of which adversely affect health (WHO, 2011b).

Gender is inextricable from the social and structural determinants shaping health and equity. Health issues differ between women and men beyond sexual and reproductive health. Biological distinctions are not enough to explain different health outcomes between men and women. Shaped by gender norms, roles and relations, there are often differences between men and women in (see Table 1) (WHO, 2011b):

- Exposure to risk factors or vulnerability;
- Household-level investment in nutrition, care and education;
- Access to and use of health services;
- Experiences in health-care settings;
- Social impacts of ill health.

Table 1 Examples of how gender norms, roles and relations influence health and contribute to health inequities

	Definitions	Examples
Gender norms	Refers to beliefs about women and men, boys and girls that are passed from generation to generation through the process of socialization. They change over time and differ in different cultures, contexts and populations. Gender norms can shape inequality if they reinforce: • Mistreatment or oppression of one group or sex over the other; or • Differences in power and opportunities.	Gender norms that associate masculinity with risk-taking and a disregard of pain and injury may lead to hazardous action by men and boys on roads. As a result, men are much more likely to die or be injured in road traffic crashes. Gender norms about social mobility and access to education and information may mean that some women have more difficulty than men in accessing health-related education and information. This can undermine their ability to understand health risks, vulnerability and the signs and symptoms of illness, as well as navigate the health system and understand their entitlements.
Gender roles	Refers to what women and men, boys and girls are expected to do (in the household, community and workplace) in a given society.	Gender roles help to shape the fields in which women and men work (both formally and informally). This is sometimes refered to as a gender-based division of labour with different health effects for women and men. For example, men are more likely to work in construction and transport due to physical demands. As a result, they are more likely to be exposed to work-related injuries. Gender roles contribute to the fact that men are over represented in nearly all forms of traumatic injury. Similarly, in some societies, women tend to be responsible for household and kitchen tasks, including cooking. As a result, women are more exposed to indoor air pollution. Indoor air pollution is associated with stroke, ischaemic heart disease, chronic obstructive pulmonary disease (COPD) and lung cancer.
Gender relations	Refers to social relations between and among women and men that are based on gender norms and roles. Gender relations often create hierarchies between and among groups of men and women that can lead to unequal power relations, disadvantaging some groups over others. Refers to sociopolitical and economic relations to institutions such as the State, corporations and social movements. This requires that we look at the collective processes by which power is mobilized and exercised. It must be understood in relation to systems and processes such as racism, sexism, homophobia (e.g. discriminatory policies, etc.) which shape gender and gendered experiences.	Unequal power relations between women and men can contribute to differential vulnerabilities to certain health conditions. For example, married women account for a large proportion of people newly infected with HIV even though often their only risk factor is having unprotected sex with their husbands. Due to gender relations and other intersecting forms of oppression, women may not have the power to negotiate safe sex or they may be reluctant to raise the issue of HIV risk with their partner for fear of disrupting a relationship of trust or risking a violent reaction by their partner. Unequal power relations may also decrease women's access to and control over essential resources (such as condoms, information on preventing HIV infection, financial resources to access and use health services etc.). Indigenous women disproportionately experience poor health and lack of access to health-promoting services (both health and social services). A recent report on the health of Indigenous Peoples states Indigenous women are "often denied access to education, land property, and other economic resources" which is "compounded by structural racism and discrimination" that "make indigenous women and children particularly vulnerable to poor health."

Source: Adapted from WHO, 2011b; UN Inter-Agency Support Group on Indigenous Peoples' Issues, 2014.

Gender analysis looks at the differences between men and women in risk and exposure, health seeking behaviour, access and use of services, experiences in health care settings, treatment options and impact of ill-health. It also looks at the interaction between biological and sociocultural factors and access to and control over resources in relation to health and identifies appropriate responses to different needs. It asks critical questions to uncover multi-level causes of gender inequality shaped by gender norms, roles and relations, unequal power relations between and among groups of women and men and the intersection of gender with other contextual factors (such as ethnicity, income and age). Drawing from the WHO Gender Analysis Questions (GAQ), examples of these may include but are not limited to (WHO, 2011b):

• Who gets ill? Are risk factors for the condition different for women and men, boys and girls? How can biological or sociocultural factors explain why women, men, boy or girls are affected differently by this condition? Are there particular activities that women or men, boys or girls typically do that may increase their exposure or vulnerability to this condition? Do women and men have the resources necessary to reduce risk and vulnerability to this condition?

• What are the ways in which those affected by the condition experience it and negotiate actions to address it? For example, how do gender norms affect willingness or ability to admit being ill and to seek treatment for this condition?

• How do access to and control over resources affect the access of care? For example, are there any indirect costs related to accessing health services that may affect women and men differently?

• How do health services meet the needs of the men and women affected by this condition? For example, how are women's and men's different roles across varying contexts considered in treatment options for this condition?

• What are the predominant health and social outcomes of this condition? For example, how do the sociocultural characteristics and consequences of the condition differ between and among women and men, such as in the division of responsibilities in the household, employability, stigma or divorce?

Gender analysis can be used to assess an existing health issue, a health project, programme or policy, health research or health service delivery. Incorporating gender analysis into policy and programme review is the process of exploring how gender and gendered power relations cross cut and interact with all other social determinants to lead to health inequities between and among men and women, including men and women's differential capacities to access and benefit from health programmes. It is important that gender analysis is incorporated and considered across any stage of the programme cycle and all steps of a review process (including the Innov8 review), so that the resulting recommendations for programme improvements are gender responsive. See the Additional Reading section for WHO guidance on gender analysis.

Recognizing that the integration of gender can make health programmes more effective, WHO promotes the use of a scale to assess the gender responsiveness of existing health policies and programmes and informs revisions to make these programmes more gender responsive (WHO, 2011b). Of the five levels outlined below, only three are desirable (Levels 3-5). During the Innov8 steps, will have the chance to consider how the programme under review currently addresses gender norms, roles and relations, and how gender relates to the multidimensional nature of health equity. In Step 7 in particular, the focus is on how the programme can become more gender responsive (ideally gender specific and gender transformative).

Table 2 Gender responsive assessment scale (GRAS)

Level 1: Gender unequal	Reinforces gender inequality by upholding or reinforcing unequal gender norms, roles and relations. Privileges one sex over the other. Often leads to one sex disproportionately enjoying more opportunities and rights.
Level 2: Gender blind	Ignores gender norms, roles and relations and very often reinforces gender-based discrimination. Ignores differences in opportunity and resource allocation for men and women across the life course. Often constructed based on the principle of being "fair" by treating everyone the same (even if needs are different).
Level 3: Gender sensitive	Indicates gender awareness and acknowledges gender-related differences and/or inequalities but takes no remedial action to address them.
Level 4: Gender specific	Considers gender norms, roles and relations for women and men and how they affect access to and control over resources. Takes account of women's and men's specific needs and takes remedial action that intentionally targets and benefits a specific group of women or men to achieve certain policy or programme goals or meet certain needs.
Level 5: Gender transformative	Considers gender norms, roles and relations for women and men, and that these affect access to and control over resources. Considers women's and men's specific needs. Takes remedial action to progressively foster equal power relationships between and among women and men by transforming harmful gender norms, roles and relations and addressing the causes of gender-based health inequity. Often explicitly promotes gender equality.

In conducting gender analysis and in being gender responsive within policies and programmes, it is imperative to understand gender as intersecting with and shaped by other social stratifiers, including ethnicity, socioeconomic status, age, disability, sexual orientation, etc. In addressing the health and health needs of men, women, boys and girls, gender must be understood as relational to such aspects of identity and experience, and not treated as an isolated or static variable. Further, gender and its intersecting social stratifiers are shaped by structures and processes of power (i.e. societal institutions, socioeconomic discrimination, stigmatization) that shape health. This means that a person may simultaneously experience both privilege and disadvantage, depending on place and time. Recognizing these complexities (which equity-informed approaches seek to do), gender analysis and gender-responsive programming facilitates understanding of, and action on, the multiple factors and processes that shape the health of individuals.

Human rights-based approach

While human rights are an important end goal, over the years, considerable efforts have also been directed towards using human rights to guide tangible programmatic interventions by national governments, the United Nations system and other multilateral and bilateral health and development agencies.

This integration and operationalization of human rights commitments in practical and concrete ways has proven challenging. A UN Common Understanding of a **human rights-based approach to programming** (HRBA) was developed to support these efforts (United Nations, 2003; United Nations 2016).

A human rights-based approach to health focuses attention and provides strategies and solutions to redress inequalities, discriminatory practices (both real and perceived) and unjust power relations, which are often at the heart of inequitable health outcomes (United Nations, 2003). The approach draws its legitimacy from the principle that health is a "right". This right is enshrined in national law in different ways. It clearly defines those responsible for its progressive realization, requiring measured progress towards the fulfilment of the core principles of a right to health (which Innov8 helps to facilitate) (United Nations, 2003). An important tenet of rights-based approaches is their support for strong accountability mechanisms. Consider the below:

> "A [HRBA] to health establishes a 'circle of accountability' throughout the policy cycle, which helps to ensure that policies and programmes are responsive to the needs of health system users. In addition to accountability, a HRBA also analyses a policy cycle through a framework of human rights principles of equality and non-discrimination, participation, indivisibility and the rule of law."
>
> (United Nations, 2015).

The goal of a HRBA to health is to ensure that all health policies, strategies and programmes be designed with the objective of *progressively improving* the enjoyment of all people to the right to health and other health related human rights, (safe and potable water, sanitation, food, housing, health related information and education, and gender), amongst others (WHO & OHCHR, 2001).

In practice, this means integrating human rights principles and norms into the design, implementation, monitoring and evaluation of policies and programmes related to health (WHO, 2013b). In this way, health systems and health services become the practical expression of the obligation of "duty-bearers" (primarily States) to realize the right to health. They should be designed to ensure that "rights holders" (such as affected individuals and communities) are informed, and equipped to know and claim their rights, or to seek redress where these are not met or are violated (WHO, 2013b). This includes addressing health rights violations that result in ill health, reducing vulnerability to ill health through human rights and promoting human rights and preventing their violation through health development. In so doing, a HRBA contributes to the development of a more equitable and responsive health system (WHO, 2013b).

In working towards the goal of human rights and particularly the right to health, human rights standards and guiding principles of indivisibility, inter-relatedness, universality, non-discrimination and equality, participation and inclusion and accountability should be respected and upheld. In defining the right to health, the Committee on Economic, Social and Cultural Rights futher unpacked the key attributes of this right, noting the importance in health settings of availability, accessibility, acceptability and quality of health services as key guiding principles. An overview of these principles as they may apply to health programmes is outlined in Box 4. The principles draw from General Comments 14 and 15 of the Committee on Economic, Social and Cultural Rights (UN CESCR 2000; UN CESCR 2003), that sought to unpack the key components of a "right to health".

Box 4 Key principles of a human rights-based approach to health

A human rights-based approach

- **Non-discrimination and equality:** Health services, goods and facilities must be provided to all without discrimination. All individuals are equal as human beings and by virtue of their inherent dignity. All human beings are entitled to their human rights without discrimination of any kind on the grounds of race, colour, sex, ethnicity, age, language, religion, political or other opinion, national or social origin, disability, property, birth or other status. In the instance that development programmes cannot reach everybody at once, priority must be given to the most marginalized. Programming must help to address underlying and systemic causes of discrimination in order to further genuine and substantive equality.

- **Participation:** There must be meaningful opportunities for engagement in all phases of the programming cycle: assessment, analysis, planning, implementation, monitoring and evaluation.

- **Accountability:** Mechanisms of accountability are crucial for ensuring that the State obligations arising from the right to health are respected. Accountability compels a State to explain what it is doing and why and how it is moving, as expeditiously and effectively as possible, towards the realization of the right to health for all. The right to health can be realized and monitored through various accountability mechanisms, but at a minimum all such mechanisms must be accessible, transparent and effective.

General Comment 14

- **Availability:** Sufficient quantities of public health and health-care facilities, goods/services and programmes.

- **Accessibility:**
  - Physical accessibility – safe physical reach (especially in rural areas);
  - Information accessibility – ability to seek, receive and impart information and ideas concerning health issues and to protect health data; Accessibility also implies the right to seek, receive and impart health-related information in an accessible format (for all, including persons with disabilities);
  - Non-discrimination; and
  - Economic accessibility – financial affordability. Accessibility also implies the right to seek,

receive and impart health-related information in an accessible format (for all, including persons with disabilities).

- **Acceptability:** Respectful of medical ethics, informed consent, patient confidentiality, and cultural appropriateness. The facilities, goods and services should also respect medical ethics, and be gender and age sensitive and culturally appropriate and acceptable.

- **Quality:** Services, goods and facilities must be scientifically and medically appropriate and of good quality. This requires, in particular, trained health professionals, scientifically approved and unexpired drugs and hospital equipment, adequate sanitation and safe drinking-water.

Sources: CESCR, 2000; CESCR, 2003; WHO, 2013b; WHO, 2014.

In applying Innov8, the HRBA principle of equality and non-discrimination is a core focus of all of the steps, as this is central to efforts to leave no one behind. For example, the principles of availability, accessibility, acceptability and quality (AAAQ) are applied through the use of the Tanahashi model of effective coverage that will be discussed in Step 4. The Tanahashi framework (Tanahashi, 1978) examines programme coverage as a series of dimensions that the beneficiary population must traverse in order to reach effective coverage and obtain the expected

benefits. An additional causal and capacity analysis will help further explain and identify relevant rights and responsibilities to redress any inequities.

The principle of participation is applied in Step 6 on intersectoral action and social participation but is a cross-cutting principle throughout the process. The principle of accountability is cross cutting, with analysis continually linking to questions of effectiveness for all subpopulations, and features prominently in Step 8 on monitoring and evaluation.

Conceptual framework of the social determinants of health

There are a number of conceptual frameworks related to social determinants of health. Review team members may know some models already, for example the Dahlgren and Whitehead (1991) "policy rainbow diagram". The WHO conceptual framework of the social determinants of health is shown in Figure 2. This analytical schema describes the factors and mechanisms by which social conditions affect people's health and produce health inequities. By showing the hierarchy of social determinants, and the mechanisms through which they act to produce health inequities, review teams will be better able to identify entry points for action.

The production of health inequities is a complex social phenomena and the framework reflects this complexity. To facilitate understanding by the review team, the framework is explained step by step.

Figure 2 Conceptual framework of the social determinants of health, WHO

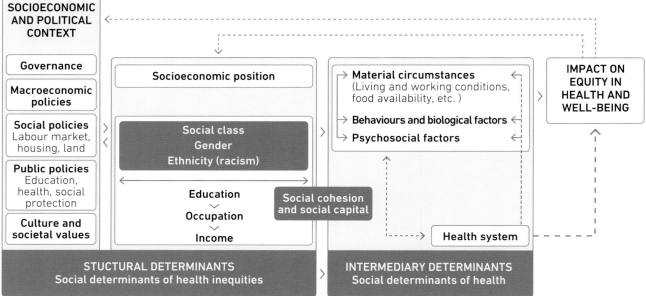

Source: Solar & Irwin, 2010.

Mechanisms of health inequities[1]

Health inequities flow from patterns of social stratification – from the systematically unequal distribution of power, prestige and resources among groups in society. It is important to consider the pathways and mechanisms through which the social determinants influence health and health inequity.

Socioeconomic position and sociocultural factors such as gender result in individuals having different levels of exposure to health-damaging conditions and differential vulnerability, in terms of health conditions and access to and control over material resources. It also contributes to individuals having differential access to health services and outcomes. Socioeconomic position (including social norms, roles and relations on gender) leads to differences in the consequences of ill health for individuals from more and less advantaged groups. These consequences include, for example, economic and social consequences (e.g. inability to work, catastrophic health expenditures, stigmatization).

Socioeconomic position influences health, *and* through the potential impact of illness on resources and prestige (i.e. through catastrophic health expenditures or stigmatization, respectively), ill health may in some contexts exert an effect on socioeconomic position and patterns of social mobility. The differential accumulation across the life course of exposures, experiences and social disadvantages that are damaging to health may widen health inequities. The social determinants of health, including gender, operate at every level of development – early childhood, childhood, adolescence and adulthood, and advanced age – both to immediately influence health and to provide the basis for health or illness

[1] This section draws considerably from Solar & Irwin (2010).

across the life course, with implications as well for the trans-generational transmission of inequities (Solar & Irwin, 2010).

For example, childhood social class will determine aspects of the early physical or psychosocial environment (e.g. exposure to air pollution or family conflict) or possible mechanisms (e.g. nutrition, infection or stress) that are associated with adult disease. Childhood social class may also influence adult health through influencing social trajectories, such as restricting educational opportunities, thus influencing socioeconomic circumstances and health in later life. Women who live longer than men are more likely to face poverty and deprivation in old age as a result of lower rates of health, education, formal employment and other disadvantage over the course of their lives. Social class during advanced age can influence levels of dependency on younger family members (usually women) to be part-time or full-time caregivers, which can in turn have implications for the income-generation activities of younger generations.

Importantly, action to address the social determinants and reduce health inequities will involve changing the distribution of power within society to benefit and empower subpopulations in situations of vulnerability and disadvantage. This requires changes to the broader socioeconomic and political context in a society to influence the relations between different subpopulations. These relations are mediated through economic, social and political institutions and mechanisms that generate, configure and maintain social hierarchies (Solar & Irwin, 2010). In this way, action on the social determinants of health inequities is a political process that engages both the agency of populations, groups and communities as well as the responsibilities of the government and other actors. Specific attention needs to be given to gendered similarities and differences when considering the mechanisms driving inequities and in the responses. Likewise, a HRBA can be useful when adjusting political processes to alter the mechanisms driving inequities

Components of the conceptual framework

Start by thinking about the health system as a social determinant of health – shown on the right of Figure 2. The health system has the responsibility to provide all people with the quality health services they need, independent of sex, ability to pay, social status or other characteristic or condition. By ensuring equitable access to health services and by promoting action across different sectors to improve health and well-being, the health system can directly influence differences in exposure and vulnerability resulting in poor health. The health system should act as a mediating force or buffer against the impacts of an

illness or disability on people's lives (Solar & Irwin, 2010). It does this by ensuring that the health problem does not result in or contribute to deterioration in a person's socioeconomic position (WHO, 2007) as well as by facilitating the social (re) integration of people with disabilities, illness or other disadvantages (Diderichsen et al, 2001; WHO, 2007).

In the conceptual framework, much of the health system (with the exception of its governance function) is represented as one of the **intermediary determinants.** These determinants are so called because – while they have important influences and impacts on health outcomes – action on them will not fundamentally affect the distribution of the power and resources in society. The governance function of health systems (including health strategies, policies and plans) is at the level of structural determinants (socioeconomic and political context).

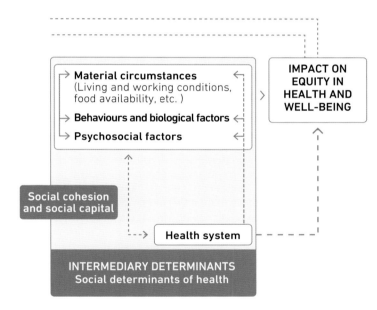

The framework shows several other categories of social determines of health, including **material circumstances**, which encompass determinants linked to material conditions including physical environments and access to social services. This includes living conditions – such as housing and neighbourhoods – and working conditions, and includes factors such as circumstances, location and the type of neighbourhood. Material circumstances also include people's ability to consume goods and services, including resources to purchase healthy foods, clothing and other necessities. These circumstances become resources that facilitate access to conditions conducive to health or alternatively constitute health risks. Gender inequities in society can manifest at this level by, for instance, differences in exposure to risk factors due to gender roles (e.g. exposure to indoor smoke due to cooking fires).

Behaviour patterns include smoking, diet, alcohol consumption and exercise. Depending on the pattern of exposure and vulnerability, behaviours may act as protective factors or enhance health (e.g. exercise and eating well) or be harmful to health (e.g. cigarette smoking and obesity). Importantly these behaviours and lifestyles are the result of material circumstances in which one is born, lives and works. They are the way that different subpopulations translate the material conditions of life into patterns of behaviour. At this level, gender norms can influence behaviour (for instance about masculinity or being "tough", which can make men and boys more likely to engage in risk-taking behaviour or postpone treatment) (WHO, 2011b).

Psychosocial factors are another category of intermediary determinants including psychosocial stressors, such as negative life events, stressful living conditions (e.g. high debt or financial insecurity) and lack of social support. Different social groups are exposed throughout their lives to different situations that are perceived as threatening, difficult to manage and/or offer little possibility for intervention (Solar & Irwin, 2010). Fear of violence (including gender-based violence), and restricted decision-making autonomy shaped by gender norms, roles and relations, are psychosocial factors that can have an impact on health (CSDH, 2007).

Related to intermediary determinants are the concepts of **social cohesion** and **social capital.** Social cohesion refers to qualities of communities and societies including having strong social relationships based on trust, a sense of inclusion (and efforts to address marginalization and exclusion) and sense of mutual obligation and respect. While there is no single definition of social capital, the key feature is that social capital refers to an intangible, dynamic and collective resource for societies that facilitates social relationships and connections. It includes elements such as trust, participation, social support and reciprocity. A high level of social cohesion and social capital works to protect people's health and well-being, including by addressing discrimination, marginalization and exclusion. Inequality can contribute to a breakdown in social cohesion and social capital.

As previously mentioned, the social determinants of health are also called intermediary determinants because they influence and impact on health outcomes, but they are not the true origins of health inequities. As the conceptual framework shows, the **social determinants of health inequities** are called **structural determinants**.

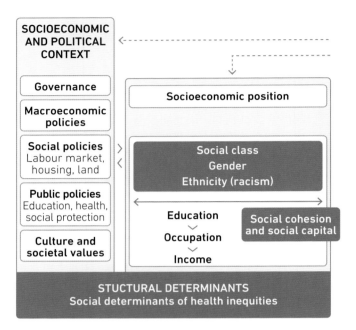

The structural determinants are the wider social, political, economic, environmental and cultural forces in society that determines people's living conditions. The key point here is that underlying the social factors that enable or constrain the health of individuals and groups are deeper societal processes that are responsible for the uneven distribution of these factors across population groups. For this reason, structural determinants are sometimes referred to as "the causes of the causes" of ill health.

Structural determinants consist of two main components, which are **socioeconomic position** and the **socioeconomic and political context**.

Socioeconomic position refers to sociocultural and economic factors that influence the position that individuals or groups have within the structure of a society. The distribution of these social and economic factors in society creates social stratification, where some individuals or groups have a higher socioeconomic position than others – this is how inequities are generated. Common factors that influence socioeconomic position include levels of income, education and occupation as well as sex, ethnicity and place of residence. The most important factors to consider, and the way they interact, vary between and among societies. As will be seen in Steps 3 and 5, differences in resources, prestige and discrimination (including based on sex, ethnicity and factors like caste) correlate with social stratification in the society.

Underlying all of the above, is the socioeconomic and political context (far left column of the framework – see Figure 2). This context is made up of a set of social, economic and political conditions in a country, which influences the equal or unequal distribution of power, resources, prestige and other social and economic factors between different groups in society. The socioeconomic and political context influences national strategies and policies related to areas such as the labour market, the educational system, social protection, and housing and land use. Gender and cultural norms are included in the social context; as stated earlier, these can manifest through discrimination when the norms imply power hierarchies, thus impacting on social stratification. The extent to which a country has ratified human rights conventions/treaties, and the strategies, policies and legal frameworks that it has in place to support progressive operationalization of human rights commitments in the national context, are an important part of the socioeconomic and political context.

Theories of evaluation and equity for health programmes

This review process draws from **theory-driven approaches to evaluation**, including **realist evaluation.** A key concept for this approach is the **programme theory**, which describes the underlying assumption on the way that the programme actions or interventions will have expected results that contribute to the achievement of programme objectives. By developing a programme theory as part of the review process, review teams will examine the assumptions of the programme more clearly and explicitly, and identify whether or not and how inequities in health, gender, human rights and social determinants of health are accounted for in the design and implementation of the health programme.

Realist evaluation places emphasis on: (i) identifying the mechanisms that produce observable effects of the programme; and (ii) testing these mechanisms and other context variables that may have impacts on the observed effects (Pawson & Tilley, 2004). It also recognizes the complexity of the transformation processes sought by programmes, and the importance of context and influence of policies and programmes from other sectors. The focus of this approach is on developing explanations of *why, where and for whom health programmes work or fail.*

Additional reading and resources

Solar O, Irwin A (2010). A conceptual framework for action on the social determinants of health. Social Determinants of Health Discussion Paper 2 (Policy and Practice). Geneva: World Health Organization. Available: http://www.who.int/sdhconference/resources/ConceptualframeworkforactiononSDH_eng.pdf, (accessed 25 February 2016).

WHO (2011b). Gender mainstreaming for health managers: a practical approach. Geneva: World Health Organization. Available: http://www.who.int/gender/documents/health_managers_guide/en/ (accessed 4 March 2016). (This reference includes the Gender Analysis Matrix and the Gender Analysis Questions.)

United Nations (2016). UN Practitioners' Portal on Human Rights Based Approaches to Programming: FAQ on HRBA. Available: http://hrbaportal.org/faq (accessed 15 June 2016).

Sridharan S, Nakaima A (2011). Ten steps to making evaluation matter. Evaluation and Program Planning. 2011;34(2):135–46. doi:10.1016/j.evalprogplan.2010.09.003.

REFERENCES

CSDH (2007). Unequal, Unfair, Ineffective and Inefficient – Gender Inequity in Health: Why it exists and how we can change it. Final Report to the WHO Commission on Social Determinants of Health. Available: http://www.who.int/social_determinants/resources/csdh_media/wgekn_final_report_07.pdf?ua=1 accessed 1 March 2016).

CSDH (2008). Closing the gap in a generation: Health equity through action on the social determinants of health. Final Report of the Commission on Social Determinants of Health. Geneva: World Health Organization. Available: http://whqlibdoc.who.int/publications/2008/9789241563703_eng.pdf?ua=1 (accessed 8 March 2016).

Dahlgren G, Whitehead M (1991). Policies and strategies to promote social equity in health. Stockholm: Institute for Future Studies.

Diderichsen F, Evans T, Whitehead M (2001). The social basis of disparities in health. In: Evans T et al, eds. Challenging inequities in health. New York: Oxford University Press.

Judge D, Stoker G, Wolman H (1998). Urban Politics and Theory: An introduction. In: Davies J, Imbroscio D, eds. Theories of Urban Politics. London: Sage Publications.

Krieger N (2001). A glossary for social epidemiology. Journal of Epidemiology and Community Health. 2001;55(10):693–700. Available: http://jech.bmj.com/content/55/10/693.full.pdf+html (accessed 4 March 2016).

Pawson R, Tilley N (2004). Realist Evaluation. London: British Cabinet Office. Available from: http://www.communitymatters.com.au/RE_chapter.pdf (accessed 18 February 2016).

Sen A (2002). Why Health Equity? Journal of Health Economics. 2002;11:659-666. Available: http://onlinelibrary.wiley.com/doi/10.1002/hec.762/pdf (accessed 29 August 2016).

Solar O, Irwin A (2010). A conceptual framework for action on the social determinants of health. Social Determinants of Health Discussion Paper 2 (Policy and Practice). Geneva: World Health Organization. Available: http://www.who.int/sdhconference/resources/ConceptualframeworkforactiononSDH_eng.pdf, (accessed 25 February 2016).

Tanahashi T (1978). Health service coverage and its evaluation. Bulletin of the World Health Organization. 1978;56(2):295–303. Available: http://www.ncbi.nlm.nih.gov/pubmed/96953 (accessed 22 February 2016).

UN CESCR (Committee on Economic, Social and Cultural Rights) (2000). General Comment No. 14: The Right to the Highest Attainable Standard of Health (Art. 12 of the Covenant), 11 August 2000, E/C.12/2000/4. Available: http://www.refworld.org/docid/4538838d0.html (accessed 4 March 2016).

UN CESCR (Committee on Economic, Social and Cultural Rights) (2003). General Comment No. 15: The Right to Water (Arts. 11 and 12 of the Covenant), 20 January 2003, E/C.12/2002/11. Available: http://www.refworld.org/docid/4538838d11.html (accessed 4 March 2016).

United Nations (2003). UN Practitioners' Portal on Human Rights Based Approaches to Programming: The Human Rights Based Approach to Development Cooperation: Towards a Common Understanding Among UN Agencies. Available: http://hrbaportal.org/the-human-rights-based-approach-to-development-cooperation-towards-a-common-understanding-among-un-agencies (accessed 4 March 2016).

United Nations (2015). Summary reflection guide on a human rights-based approach to health. Application to sexual and reproductive health, maternal health and under-5 child health. National Human Rights Institutions. Geneva. Available: http://www.ohchr.org/Documents/Issues/Women/WRGS/Health/RGuide_NHRInsts.pdf (accessed 4 March 2016).

United Nations (2016). UN Practitioners' Portal on Human Rights Based Approaches to Programming: FAQ on HRBA. Available: http://hrbaportal.org/faq (accessed 15 June 2016).

UN Inter-Agency Support Group on Indigenous Peoples' Issues (2014). The Health of Indigenous Peoples. Thematic Paper on the Health of Indigenous Peoples. Available: http://www.un.org/en/ga/president/68/pdf/wcip/IASG%20Thematic%20Paper%20-%20Health%20-%20rev1.pdf (accessed 7 March 2016).

WHA (2009). World Health Assembly Resolution 62.14: Reducing health inequities through action on the SDH. Geneva: World Health Organization. Available: http://apps.who.int/gb/ebwha/pdf_files/WHA62-REC1/WHA62_REC1-en.pdf (accessed 22 February 2016).

WHA (2012). World Health Assembly Resolution 65.8: Outcome of the World Health Conference on Social Determinants of Health. Geneva: World Health Organization. Available: http://www.who.int/sdhconference/background/A65_R8-en.pdf?ua=1 (accessed 22 February 2016).

Whitehead M (1991). The concepts and principles of equity and health. Health Promotion International. 1991;6(3):217–228.

WHO (1946). Constitution of the World Health Organization. New York. Available: http://apps.who.int/gb/bd/PDF/bd47/EN/constitution-en.pdf (accessed 4 March 2016).

WHO (2007). Everybody's business: Strengthening health systems to improve health outcomes. WHO's framework for action. Geneva: World Health Organization. Available: http://www.who.int/healthsystems/strategy/everybodys_business.pdf (accessed 4 March 2016)

WHO (2011a). Closing the gap: Policy into practice on social determinants of health. Discussion paper. Geneva: World Health Organization. Available: http://www.who.int/sdhconference/Discussion-paper-EN.pdf (accessed 24 February 2015).

WHO (2011b). Gender mainstreaming for health managers: a practical approach. Geneva: World Health Organization. Available: http://www.who.int/gender/documents/health_managers_guide/en/ (accessed 4 March 2016).

WHO (2011c) Rio Political Declaration on Social Determinants of Health. Rio de Janeiro: Brazil. Available: http://www.who.int/sdhconference/declaration/Rio_political_declaration.pdf?ua=1 (accessed 22 February 2016).

WHO (2013a). WHO (2013). Demonstrating a health in all policies analytic framework for learning from experiences: based on literature reviews from Africa, South-East Asia and the Western Pacific. Geneva: World Health Organization. Available: http://apps.who.int/iris/bitstream/10665/104083/1/9789241506274_eng.pdf (accessed 7 March 2016).

WHO (2013b). Women's and children's health: Evidence of impact of human rights. Bustreo F, Hunt P, eds. Geneva: World Health Organization. Available: http://apps.who.int/iris/bitstream/10665/84203/1/9789241505420_eng.pdf?ua=1 (accessed 4 March 2016).

WHO (2014). Ensuring human rights in the provision of contraceptive information and services: Guidance and recommendations. Geneva: World Health Organization. Available: http://apps.who.int/iris/bitstream/10665/102539/1/9789241506748_eng.pdf?ua=1 (accessed 4 March 2016).

WHO and OHCHR (2001). Factsheet No. 31. The Right to Health. Geneva. Available: http://www.who.int/hhr/activities/Right_to_Health_factsheet31.pdf (accessed 4 March 2016).

WHO Regional Office for Europe (1990). The concepts and principles of equity and health. (Whitehead M, document number: EUR/ICP/RPD 414). Copenhagen: WHO Regional Office for Europe. Available: http://salud.ciee.flacso.org.ar/flacso/optativas/equity_and_health.pdf (accessed 4 March 2016).

World Health Organization Regional Office for Europe (2006). Concepts and principles for tackling social inequities in health. (Whitehead M, Dahlgren G). Copenhagen: WHO Regional Office for Europe. Available: http://www.euro.who.int/__data/assets/pdf_file/0010/74737/E89383.pdf (accessed 4 March 2016).

Step1

Complete the
diagnostic checklist

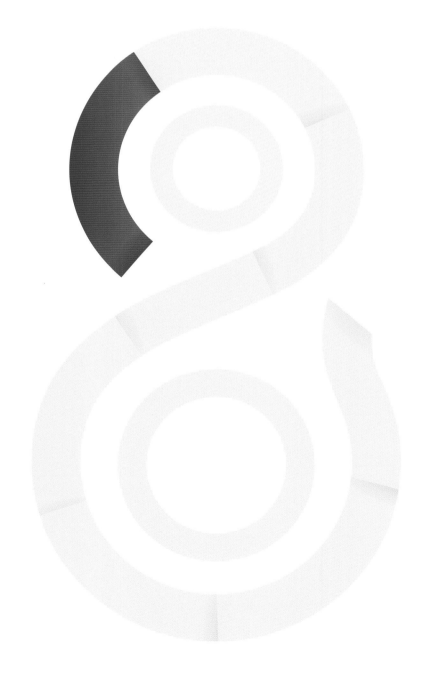

Overview

In Step 1 the review team will complete an initial assessment of the health programme using a diagnostic checklist. The report that emerges is a baseline that reflects the current situation for the programme, and includes a preliminary assessment of challenges related to equity, gender, human rights and social determinants of health. Checklist findings are useful on their own, but they are also drawn from for subsequent steps.

The checklist consists of questions on the programme's objectives, structure, organization, process of planning, implementation, monitoring and evaluation. Some questions involve concepts and principles covered in the previous chapter, which review team members should read before starting Step 1.

An overview of the checklist questions is provided in Box 1.1 of this chapter. The checklist questions are not meant to be prescriptive nor answered mechanically. Rather, they should be examined through the specific country and programmatic lens. If needed, national adaptations are encouraged. Any adaptations, however, should maintain the essential nature of the question, as answers inform the subsequent steps of the Innov8 process. Ideally, adjustments should be documented and shared with WHO to facilitate follow up and learning across contexts.

Step 1 fosters teamwork by providing guided spaces for reflective discussions on the programme, so that team members are able to reach deliberative consensus. Completing the checklist reinforces the review team's commitment to developing a critical and constructive analysis of the programme.

In answering questions, the review team should draw on programme documents (such as programme reports or past evaluations) and other information gathered, and cite these where appropriate. In some countries, review teams have benefited by engaging other professionals, including health information and statistics departments and national statistics institutes, when responding to the questions. For this reason it is important to include the local programme operators (such as primary care providers) and civil society organizations and representatives from other sectors. The team may also wish to consult with other actors.

The main output of Step 1 is the completed diagnostic checklist template and a short report summarizing the findings and conclusions.

Objectives of Step 1

> Complete a diagnostic checklist to identify and describe key aspects of the programme's objectives, structure, organization, process of planning, implementation, monitoring and evaluation.

> Develop preliminary reflections on the potential equity, gender, human rights and social determinants of health issues to be developed in the review and redesign proposal.

COMPLETE THE DIAGNOSTIC CHECKLIST
STEP 1

Box 1.1 Overview of the checklist questions

1. What are the stated goal(s), objectives and expected outcomes of the programme?
   a. What are the goal(s) and objectives of the programme?
   b. What are the expected results of the programme?
   c. Is there a specific objective on leaving no one behind in the programme (see explanation on equity, gender, human rights and social determinants)?

2. What is the topic or problem that the programme addresses?

3. How are human rights, including the right to health, incorporated in the health programme?
   a. Do the review team and other people working on the programme consider human rights in relation to the programme?
   b. How does documentation on the programme refer to international human rights, treaties, conventions or standards on the right to health including concluding observations or recommendations?

4. What is the target population of the programme and are any subpopulations prioritized?
   a. What is the programme's target population?
   b. Does the programme define any priority subpopulations within the target population(s)?
   c. For the above subpopulations, does the programme consider how social characteristics and gender norms, roles and relations influence each subpopulation?

5. How does the programme assess population needs?
   a. How does the programme assess population needs?
   b. How does the programme assess the differential needs of specific subpopulations (including those linked to gender norms, roles and relations)?

6. What are the main interventions, services or activities of the programme?
   a. What are the interventions, services or activities of the programme?
   b. What implementation difficulties have been identified for the above set of programme interventions?

7. How do the programme interventions, services and activities consider context?
   a. How do the interventions, services and activities consider the contexts within which the target population(s) live?
   b. How are interventions, services and activities differentiated for any subpopulations?

8. Who implements or carries out the interventions?
   a. Who implements or carries out the interventions (e.g. subnational and local providers)?
   b. How do implementers participate in the planning, monitoring, review and evaluation?

9. How does the programme incorporate principles of a human rights-based approach including non-discrimination and equality, participation, accountability, as well as elements of the right to health (availability, accessibility, acceptability and quality)?

10. How does the programme include mechanisms for social participation?
    a. What groups or organizations participate and through which mechanisms?
    b. What are the main challenges for social participation?

11. How does the programme include intersectoral action?
    a. Please indicate how the programme includes intersectoral action.
    b. What are the main challenges and difficulties for carrying out intersectoral work?

12. What are the main achievements of this programme and what indicators does the programme use to verify these?
    a. What are the main results and achievements of the programme?
    b. What indicators does the programme use to verify achievements?
    c. What equity, gender, human rights or social determinants indicators, if any, does the programme use to verify achievements or track in relation to the programme?
    d. How does the programme carry out programme review and evaluation? Who participates and how often?

13. What are some of the potential equity, gender, human rights and social determinants of health issues to be addressed in the review?

Source: Adapted from the original diagnostic checklist developed by the Government of Chile (Ministerio de Salud, Chile, 2010:30).

CHECKLIST TEMPLATE

The review team should use this template to answer the checklist questions. Any national adaptations or changes should be specified. It is recommended that the review team prepare a brief narrative report (three to four pages) summarizing the main findings and appending the completed checklist template.

Date or response period

Official programme name (include name in national language and English translation)

Institution where the programme is based

Names of team members who worked on the checklist	Role in relation to the programme or, if you are not programme staff, your affiliation (e.g. from another part of the ministry, civil society organization, research institute, national human rights institutions, parliamentarians)
1.	1.
2.	2.
3.	3.
4.	4.
5.	5.
6.	6.
7.	7.
8	8

COMPLETE THE DIAGNOSTIC CHECKLIST
STEP 1

1. What are the stated goal(s), objectives and expected outcomes of the programme?

The objectives and expected outcomes should be specific to the programme or intervention package rather than to the health system in general.

A **programme goal** is a broad statement describing the long-term, ultimate aim of the programme. It serves as the foundation for developing the

programme objectives. **Programme objectives** describe the results to be achieved and how they will be achieved. **Expected results** are outcomes that a programme is designed to produce.

1.a. What are the goal(s) and objectives of the programme? Please list them.

```



```

1.b. What are the expected results of the programme? Please list them.

```



```

1.c. Is there a specific objective on leaving no one behind in the programme (see explanation on equity, gender, human rights and social determinants)? If yes, please describe it.

This type of **objective** should specifically seek the reduction or elimination of health differences among subpopulations that are systematic and avoidable.

Objectives may draw on selected aspects related to equity, social determinants of health, gender-responsive and human rights-based approaches in ways that enhance health equity. For instance, an objective may aim to reduce or eliminate avoidable and unfair differences shaped by gender norms, roles and relations, or it may aim to ensure non-discrimination and equality in keeping with a human rights-based approach.

Although a universal coverage objective seeks to meet the needs of all groups, in itself it does not necessarily constitute an objective focused on leaving no one behind. This is because, in reforms towards UHC, specific efforts are needed to ensure that these reforms benefit more disadvantaged subpopulations as least as much as more advantaged subpopulations. The rationale is that there may be barriers that prevent more disadvantaged subpopulations from fully benefitting from universal coverage reforms, and objectives to leave no one behind specifically address those barriers. However, measures targeting certain marginalized subpopulations only (disregarding a wider universal coverage approach) are also not conducive to the objective of leaving no one behind in relation to the SDGs, which have as one of their targets Universal Health Coverage.

COMPLETE THE DIAGNOSTIC CHECKLIST
STEP 1

2. What is the topic or problem that the programme addresses?

The topic or problem addressed by the programme, sometimes called the **problem space** (Sridharan, 2012), describes the issues of interest related to the problem contemplated in the programme – what factors are associated with it, how that problem changes over time and ideally how it is distributed within the population. The problem space may or may not consider health inequities. For example, health programmes may: seek to prevent, treat or address a particular disease or disorder (e.g. tuberculosis, hypertension, mental health); target a particular risk factor (e.g. tobacco, unhealthy food, air pollution); focus on a particular body system (e.g. cardiovascular, respiratory); or focus on health across the life course (e.g. adolescent health), among other types of classification.

What is the topic or problem that the programme addresses?

3. How are human rights, including the right to health, incorporated in the health programme?

3.a. **Do the review team and other people working on the programme consider human rights in relation to the programme? Please describe your concrete experience on human rights in, for example, the programme cycle and day-to-day work.**

3.b. How does documentation on the programme refer to international human rights, treaties, conventions or standards on the right to health including concluding observations and recommendations? Please specify how human rights are referred to and operationalized in the programme.

This question is asking if the programme makes reference to standards enshrined in any of the international human rights treaties, conventions or standards on the right to health in programme documentation. These include the UN Convention on the Rights of the Child (CRC); Convention on the Elimination of All Forms of Discrimination against Women (CEDAW); UN Convention on the Rights of Persons with Disabilities (CRPD); and the International Covenant on Economic, Social and Cultural Rights (ICESCR). If the programme does not expressly refer to the human rights treaties, conventions or standards – which may be the case – this should be noted.

---

4. What is the target population of the programme and are any subpopulations prioritized?

The following list of subpopulations may be useful to help the review team answer this question, but other subpopulations relevant for the specific programme and context should also be included.

4.a. What is the programme's target population?

Please include the **programme statement** of the target population (including an estimation of population size in absolute numbers and percentage of the total population, and if both women and men, or girls and boys are included).

4.b. Does the programme define any priority subpopulations within the target population(s)? If yes, indicate which subpopulations and why are they prioritized?

Provide an explanation. Review the following list of specific subpopulations and tick those that apply.

Indicate if any of the following subpopulations are prioritized	Tick any relevant
Targeted based on sex	
Age-related groups (e.g. children, youth, seniors, etc.)	
Disability (e.g. physical, deaf, visual, intellectual/developmental, learning, mental illness, addictions/substance use, etc.)	
Ethno-racial communities (e.g. aboriginal/indigenous groups, racial or cultural minorities, etc.)	
High risk groups for exposure to specific risk factors	
Income or education groups	
Persons with specific occupations or employment status (e.g. employed in the informal sector, under-employed or unemployed, or in occupations like sex work, mining)	
Persons of migrant, asylum seeker and refugee status (including regular, irregular, internal migrant)	
Religious/faith communities	
Populations in rural/remote areas or disadvantaged urban areas (e.g. geographic or social isolation, under-serviced areas, etc.)	
Other: please describe the subpopulation here	

4.c. For the above subpopulations, how does the programme consider how social characteristics and gender norms, roles and relations influence each subpopulation? Please give a short explanation.

5. How does the programme assess population needs?

5.a. How does the programme assess population needs?
If there is a needs assessment for the programme, please attach the document.

Health programmes should be based on an assessment of the needs of the population, in relation to the health issue the programme is addressing. This informs what, how and to whom interventions, services or activities are provided. Population needs can be assessed in different ways. In many health programmes, the needs of the population are defined by **experts (such as doctors or policy-makers), often according to standards, norms or criteria**. There are other ways, however, to assess population need. One way is **asking people through surveys or consultation** about their perceived needs (i.e. their problems or expectations). Another way is to assess

the need that is "expressed" by people through their **actions and demand for services** in relation to the health issue. This assessment is often based on information about the use of health services from health service registers and waiting lists. A final way to assess population needs is to **compare with groups** who have characteristics similar to those who receive services, as a way to assess needs in terms of gaps in health service coverage (Bradshaw, 1972).

This question is asking you to indicate **who** makes the decisions about the programme needs, and **what information** their decisions are based on, in terms of the above ways of assessing needs.

5.b. How does the programme assess the differential needs of specific subpopulations?

For example, has a gender analysis been done as part of the needs assessment? Does the needs assessment consider how gender influences women's and men's differential exposure to risks, household-level investment in nutrition, care and education, access to and use of services, experiences in health care settings, health outcomes and social consequences of ill-health? This type of analysis identifies differences between men/boys and women/girls, due to: (i) gender norms, roles, and relations; (ii) differential access to and control over resources; and (iii) biological (e.g. sex-based) differences, across the life course.

Looking at differential needs should not be limited to considering sex and gender only; it is important to also consider other social stratifiers such as place of residence (rural/urban), income level and education, among others, as well as their linkages (since many have a role in shaping and/or being shaped by others).

6. What are the main interventions, services or activities of the programme?

6.a. What are the interventions, services or activities of the programme? List them and categorize them in the following table.

A programme "intervention, service or activity" refers to an action that enables attainment of one or more of the programme objectives, and hence serves to deliver the expected results. These can be delivered to **individuals** or they can be **population based**. For example, prenatal interventions and neonatal services are individual interventions. Examples of population interventions, which act on population-level determinants to change the social context that influences health, are cigarette taxes or smoking bans in public places, fortification of foods like flour and milk, and environmental health regulations.

Some confusion may arise in relation to the terms **population** and **universal**. A programme may have universal coverage for individual interventions, but this does not always signify that it is a population-based intervention. Universal coverage of all people with a specific need for an individualized treatment may not produce population impact. Nevertheless, in some cases, such as immunization, universal coverage results in positive externalities even for those not immunized (herd effect). For this reason, some experts refer to immunization as a population intervention.

Programme interventions/services/activities	Is the intervention individual or population based? (Tick the column that applies)	
	Individual	Population based
1.		
2.		
3.		
4.		
5.		

6.b. What implementation difficulties have been identified for the above set of programme interventions? Please describe these.

Examples of implementation difficulties include: deficits in the availability of adequately skilled health professionals, problems of quality, unavailability of inputs like medicines and technologies, acceptability of services, lack of or delayed expression of health need by target population and/or problems with adherence to treatment by patients, distance from health facilities (combined with lack of transportation or transportation costs) for members of the target population.

7. How do the programme interventions, services and activities consider context?

7.a. How do the interventions, services and activities consider the contexts within which the target population(s) live?

7.b. How are interventions, services and activities differentiated for any subpopulations?

For example, how do they consider the population's living and working conditions, or discrimination (for instance, based on ethnicity, class, sex, gender identity and sexual orientation)? Was the context of men's and/or women's lives and their different health needs considered? How have gender norms, roles and relations and other cultural norms been taken into account?

8. Who implements or carries out the interventions?

a) Who implements or carries out the interventions (e.g. subnational and local providers)? For each intervention described above, list the implementers.	b) How do implementers participate in the planning, monitoring, review and evaluation?
1.	
2.	
3.	
4.	
5.	

9. How does the programme incorporate the following principles of a human rights-based approach and elements of the right to health?

How does the programme incorporate/address the following principles of a human rights-based approach and elements of the right to health?
See *Introduction to applied concepts, principles and frameworks* for an explanation of each.

- **Non-discrimination and equality**
- **Participation**
- **Accountability**
- **Availability**
- **Accessibility**
- **Acceptability**
- **Quality**

10. How does the programme include mechanisms for social participation?

10.a. What groups or organizations participate and through which mechanisms?

10.b. What are the main challenges for social participation (based on the review team's knowledge and experience)?

11. How does the programme include intersectoral action?

11.a. Please indicate how the programme includes intersectoral action, by completing the following table.

Sector	What are you doing with this sector?	What is the purpose or objective of working together?
Education		
Social planning		
Social protection		
Women's affairs		
Labour		
Housing		
Agriculture		
Financing		
Other (please add)		

11.b. What are the main challenges and difficulties for carrying out intersectoral work (based on the review team's knowledge and experience)?

COMPLETE THE DIAGNOSTIC CHECKLIST
STEP 1

12. What are the main achievements of this programme and what indicators does the programme use to verify these?

In answering the below questions, please cite any relevant programme documents, and ensure that they are included in the compendium of data sources and information.

12.a. What are the main results and achievements of the programme?

12.b. What indicators does the programme use to verify achievements?

The programme may have a variety of performance indicators across the results chain of inputs, processes, outputs, outcomes and impacts. For example, does the programme have any **impact indicators** (e.g. measurable changes in quality of life, reduced incidence of diseases, increased income for women, reduced mortality)? Does the programme have **process indicators**, which are those that measure the progress of activities in a programme/ project and the way these are carried out (e.g. referring to the degree of participation or sometimes including the input indicators like the quantity, quality and timeliness of resources such as human, financial and material, technological and information) for a programme or activity (adapted from Patton, 1997: 220)?

12.c. What equity, gender, human rights or social determinants indicators, if any, does the programme use to verify achievements or track in relation to the programme?

These indicators include those that allow for equity stratification of other indicators, in relation for instance to coverage rates, morbidity and mortality by sex, place of residence (rural/urban), income, education or other relevant stratifiers for the national context. They may also touch on issues such as, but not limited to, perceived experiences of discrimination by treatment providers, reasons for not seeking care (e.g. linked to need to request permission, financial barriers, distance barriers), and experiences with participation in programme design, planning, implementation, monitoring and evaluation. Indicators can also aim to monitor progress on gender equality, including measures on empowerment (of women and of the community), or process and outcome indicators for gender mainstreaming.

12.d. How does the programme carry out programme review and evaluation? Who participates and how often?

COMPLETE THE DIAGNOSTIC CHECKLIST
STEP 1

13. After completing the checklist and drawing on the team's experience and knowledge, what are some of the potential equity, gender, human rights and social determinants of health issues to be addressed in the review?

Equity

Gender

Human rights

Social determinants of health

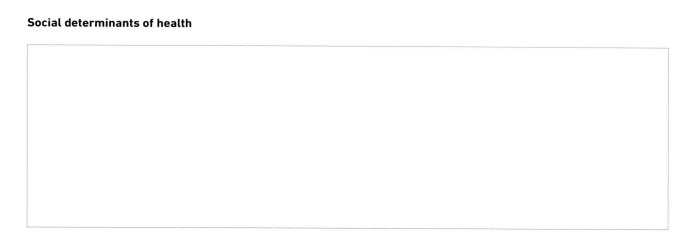

Remember that these conclusions about the main challenges are preliminary and will continue to develop as the review team continues with the next steps of the review.

REFERENCES

Bradshaw J (1972). A taxonomy of social need. In: Mclachlan G, ed. Problems and progress in medical care: essays on current research. 7th series. Oxford: Nuffield Provincial Hospital Trust.

Ministerio de Salud, Chile (2010). Documento Técnico II: Pauta para Iniciar la Revisión de los Programas: Lista de Chequeo de Equidad. Serie de Documentos Técnicos del Rediseño de los Programas desde la Perspectiva de Equidad y Determinantes Sociales. Santiago: Subsecretaría de Salud Pública. [Ministry of Health, Chile (2010). Technical document II for supporting the review and redesign of public health programmes from the perspective of equity and social determinants of health. Santiago: Undersecretary for Public Health.] Materials in Spanish only.

Ministry of Health, Social Services and Equality, Spain (2012). Methodological guide to integrate equity into health strategies, programmes and activities. Version 1. Madrid. Available: http://www.msssi.gob.es/profesionales/saludPublica/prevPromocion/promocion/desigualdadSalud/jornadaPresent_Guia2012/docs/Methodological_Guide_Equity_SPAs.pdf (accessed 17 February 2016).

Patton QM (1997). Utilization focused evaluation: The new century text. 3rd edition. London: Sage Publications.

Sridharan S (2012). A Pocket Guide to Evaluating Health Equity Interventions – Some Questions for Reflection by Sanjeev Sridharan. Magic: Measuring & Managing Access Gaps in Care (blog entry). Available: http://www.longwoods.com/blog/a-pocket-guide-to-evaluating-health-equity-interventions-some-questions-for-reflection/ (accessed 17 February 2016).

Additional resources consulted in formulating this checklist

CDC (2013). A Practitioner's Guide for Advancing Health Equity: Community Strategies for Preventing Chronic Disease. Atlanta, Georgia: Centers for Disease Control and Prevention. Available: http://www.cdc.gov/nccdphp/dch/health-equity-guide/index.htm (accessed 17 February 2016).

Government of Tasmania (2016). Equity Checklist. Web page. Department of Health and Human Resources. Available: http://www.dhhs.tas.gov.au/healthpromotion/wihpw/principles/equity/checklist_equity (accessed 17 February 2016).

Ontario Public Health Association (2010). Health equity checklist reference document. Available: http://opha.on.ca/OPHA/media/Resources/Resource%20Documents/Health_Equity_Checklist-Reference_Document.pdf?ext=.pdf (accessed 17 February 2016).

Pauly B, MacDonald M, O'Briain W, Hancock T, Perkin K, Martin W, Zeisser C, Lowen C, Wallace B, Beveridge R, Cusack E, Riishede J, on behalf of the ELPH Research Team (2013). Health Equity Tools. Victoria, BC: University of Victoria. Available: http://www.uvic.ca/research/projects/elph/assets/docs/Health%20Equity%20Tools%20Inventory.pdf (accessed 17 February 2016).

Sudbury and District Health Unit (2014). Health equity mapping checklist. Government of Canada.

University of York (2011). An equity checklist: a framework for health technology assessments. Centre for Health Economics Research Paper 62. Available: http://www.york.ac.uk/media/che/documents/papers/researchpapers/CHERP62_an_equity_checklist_a_framework_for_HTA_.pdf (accessed 17 February 2016).

COMPLETE THE DIAGNOSTIC CHECKLIST
STEP 1

USAID (2010). Equity framework for health. Policy brief from Health Policy Initiative, Task Order 1. Available: http://www.healthpolicyinitiative.com/index.cfm?ID=topicEquity (accessed 17 February 2016).

USAID and Maternal and Child Health Integrated Program (2013). Checklist for Health Equity Programming. Washington DC. Available: http://www.mchip.net/sites/default/files/Checklist%20for%20MCHIP%20Health%20Equity%20Programming_FINAL_formatted%20_2_.pdf (accessed 17 February 2016).

WHO (2011). Human rights and gender equality in health sector strategies: How to assess policy coherence. Geneva: World Health Organization. Available: http://www.ohchr.org/Documents/Publications/HRandGenderEqualityinHealthSectorStrategies.pdf (accessed 17 February 2016).

WHO (2013). Women's and children's health: Evidence of impact of human rights. Geneva: World Health Organization. Available: http://apps.who.int/iris/bitstream/10665/84203/1/9789241505420_eng.pdf?ua=1 (accessed 17 February 2016).

Step2

Understand the
programme theory

Overview

In Step 2, the review team focuses on understanding and articulating how and why the programme's interventions and activities are expected to produce results; in other words, the "programme theory".

The programme's purpose or objective is not the same as the programme theory. Rather the programme theory describes *how the programme activities are understood to contribute to a series of outputs and outcomes that should lead to the intended longer term impacts*. The programme theory is very similar to the evaluative concept of a "theory of change", but applied specifically to a programme.

The programme theory is often not explicit, so it needs to be "uncovered" by the review team. The five activities of Step 2 guide the review team towards articulating the programme theory, by means of:

1) Developing a better understanding of the health problem that the programme addresses;

2) Examining the interventions that make up the programme's response to the problem in order to produce a positive change for the target population;

3) Illustrating, through a flow diagram, the main programme components (key stages), including the interventions or groups of activities, outputs, outcomes and impacts;

4) Writing a programme theory statement that explains what has to happen for the outcomes to be met and sets out the assumptions about why; and

5) Considering whether the current programme theory explicitly considers equity, gender, human rights and social determinants of health.

In completing the activities, the review team will draw on the findings from Step 1 as well as the programme documents and information gathered.

The main output of Step 2 is a statement on the programme theory and a logic model diagram of the programme's key stages. The understanding of the current programme theory is the starting point for examining how the programme works in practice and for whom it works or fails and why; it is tested in the steps that follow. The same programme may work or fail for different subpopulations in different conditions, generating inequities if the heterogeneities and varying contexts are not considered.

___

Objectives of Step 2

> Identify the general characteristics of the programme, including the components or key stages, the specific activities, and the expected results.

> Develop a logic model diagram of the key stages of the programme, which depicts the flow of interventions or groups of activities, outputs and expected results.

> Apply theory-driven concepts to understand the logic model of the programme and the underlying assumptions about population engagement and context.

> Determine how the programme addresses equity, gender, human rights and social determinants and considers different contexts, the heterogeneity of subpopulations and the complexity of the interventions.

> Write a statement of the current theory of the programme.

BACKGROUND READING FOR STEP 2

This background reading and the additional readings aim to provide conceptual orientations to the review team for understanding programme theory:

• Moving from a "problem space" to a "solution space";

• The theory of a programme (starting with its "ABC");

• Building a diagram of the key stages of the programme and a statement of its theory; and

• Assessing if and how the programme theory includes measures to address equity, gender, human rights and social determinants of health.

Moving from a "problem space" to a "solution space"

Interventions to improve health equity are often implemented without clarity about the underlying mechanisms generating the inequities. Understanding these mechanisms underlying intervention aimed at improving health and health inequities requires clarifying how the programme is likely to work and for whom in a given context. This awareness, in turn,

will support the identification of how and when equity, gender, human rights and social determinants of health could be better integrated into each programme intervention or activity. To do this requires a shift from considering the problem space to a stronger focus on the solution space, as outlined in Box 2.1.

Box 2.1 The problem space and the solution space

"It is useful to differentiate between evidence of the 'problem space' and evidence for the 'solution space'. The 'problem space' provides knowledge of what variables or systems of relationships are associated with health inequities (e.g. information on gradients of health inequities) while the 'solution space' offers knowledge of what kinds of interventions are likely to 'work', 'for whom' and under what contexts. Much of the research on health inequities to date has focused on the

problem space of health inequities. The 'solution space' has not received the attention in the literature it most certainly deserves. Existing knowledge of the 'solution space' is often incomplete for the successful implementation of interventions in specific settings. For example, 'off the shelf' literature on best practices does not often provide information on the contexts necessary for the programme to work."

Sridharan, 2012.

The theory of a programme: Conceptualizing the problem(s) and examining the programme's interventions and activities

Health programmes are complex by nature, often aiming to tackle a set of related problems or issues at once in an open system with multiple contextual influences, which in turn makes evaluating the programme a complex process. Theory-based

evaluation approaches, including the realist perspective, suggest that articulating the logic of interventions and taking into account the mechanisms through which they produce the outcomes in a specific context – the theory of the programme – helps to inform this undertaking. This approach focuses on the configuration of context-mechanism-outcomes (Lacouture et al, 2015)

To understand the programme theory, it is first important to understand what the programme is designed to achieve. That is, what problem or issue the programme is seeking to influence and what actions are taken because they are assumed to have particular expected effects. Analysing the programme's organization, interventions and activities, and lines of actions will help in identifying the assumptions behind the actions, i.e. "if we do action A ... we expect that outcome B will happen because ...". The programme theory is described in Box 2.2.

Box 2.2 The theory of a programme

The theory of a programme can be described as **the representation of the mechanisms by which means it is understood that the programme activities contribute to the expected outcomes, in the short, medium and long term**. It is a model that specifies what must be done to achieve the objectives, and to understand what actually happens in each key stage of the programme (Rogers, 2000).

Since programmes are always introduced into pre-existing social contexts, these prevailing conditions interact with the programme mechanisms to determine the successes and failures. Including assumptions about the interactions with contextual factors are part of a comprehensive understanding of the workings of the programme (Pawson & Tilley, 1997).

A useful starting point for understanding the programme theory is to identify what Pawson and Sridharan (2009) call the **"ABC" of the programme**. This includes:

A. **Conceptualization and contextualization of the problem to be addressed:** Contextualization of the problem (whether it is a social, institutional or environmental problem) refers to where the health problem occurs and the causal model of the health problem.

B. **What to do:** The changes that must occur to address, reduce or eliminate these problems in the specific context.

C. **How to do it:** The actions that are required to bring about new solutions and resources to individuals or communities facing the health problem, so as to bring about the changes the programme aims at and on which it is based (mechanisms).

In simple terms, the ABC is the response to the question: Why does the programme's existence make a difference?

Building a diagram of the key stages of the programme

Identifying the programme ABC and the types of interventions and intervention coverage gives the review team information necessary to develop a programme diagram. A programme diagram is a visual representation or a logic model that shows the key stages of the programme required to reach the intended change or outcome, and how these stages are organized and sequenced.

Figure 2.1 is an example of a programme diagram for "Have a Heart Paisley", which was a national demonstration project in Scotland aimed at reducing coronary heart disease (CHD) in the town of Paisley. The diagram depicts the theory underlying the organization of the programme and its interventions to produce the expected outcomes.

Figure 2.1 Have a Heart Paisley

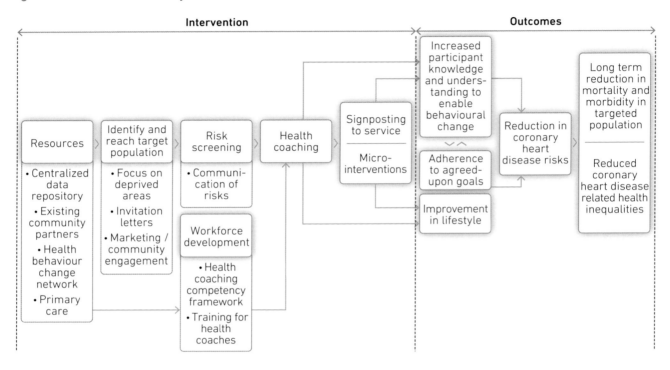

Sources: Sridharan et al, 2008:8; Sridharan, 2009.

The idea of causation is central to a programme diagram. The **logic model approach** may be useful for this purpose (Taylor-Powell & Henert, 2008). A logic model illustrates a programme's assumed causal connections. However, this representation may be challenging to depict because, as Taylor-Powell and Henert (2008: Handout 12 "About Causation", with adaptations by authors) identify, the evidence shows that:

- In almost all cases, programmes have only a partial influence over results. Contexts (external factors) beyond the programme's control influence the flow of events. This applies particularly to longer term outcomes.

- The strength of contextual influences that affect the development and implementation of the programme make it difficult to tease out causal connections. Each social group has specific characteristics and are embedded in a web of influences that affect health outcomes (living and working conditions, family relationships, experiences, economy, culture, etc.). The context affects the programme, and at the same time the context is also affected by the programme.

- Seldom is there a single cause. There are more likely multiple cause-effect chains that interact.

- Data collected through various methods – quantitative and qualitative – often show different causal associations. Rarely is it proved that a particular outcome is the result of a particular intervention.

- Causal relationships are usually not simple or clear. Rather, there are multiple and interacting relationships that affect change, often functioning as feedback loops with the possibility of delays.

- Systems theory suggests a dynamic and circular approach to understanding causal relationships rather than a uni-dimensional, linear approach.

Logic models can be created to depict these more iterative, causal mechanisms and relationships by adding feedback loops and two-way arrows, narrative explanations or a matrix. Limitations are imposed by the necessity of communicating on paper in a two-dimensional space such complexity. But ultimately,

the test of a logic model is its usefulness in clarifying the programme's intervention pathways to results.

Assessing if and how the programme theory includes measures to address equity, gender, human rights and social determinants of health

Critical to assessing for whom and in what circumstances a health programme works is examining if and how the programme's interventions and activities are directed towards the reduction of inequities and to addressing the determinants of health, including discrimination based on sex, gender or ethnicity. Two important aspects to consider when examining these questions are context and the heterogeneity of the population.

Context where programme is implemented: Contexts are the contingent conditions in which the programme happens and engages with the target population. These conditions may affect the connections between the programme mechanisms and outcomes. Programme activities may have different effects on or implications for different subpopulations in the target population. Context encompasses social structures, national policies, community norms and conventions, including the role of gender, social class, income, institutional structures and cultural systems among other factors. Research repeatedly shows that contextual factors, varying from place to place and changing over time, frustrate programme efforts (Fulop & Robert, 2013).

In realistic evaluation, context becomes a main focus of an intervention, because of the close relationship between the effectiveness of interventions and the influences arising from the context in which the programme is implemented. Furthermore, while the results of interventions are context dependent, at the same time the context is modified by the interventions themselves (de Souza, 2013).

The contextual influences occur at macro, meso and micro levels. At the macro level, certain political and policy conditions shape health and social protection systems, driving policy and programme initiatives aimed at achieving greater equity, action on social determinants of health, and addressing gender and human rights issues. In turn, the macro influences

facilitate or hinder the meso or institutional level objectives of integrating the praxis of equity, gender and human rights. At the micro level of programme operators or frontline providers the quality and coherence of the programme may be constrained by local contextual factors, including the institutional culture and community resources and relationships with other actors and programmes (Fulop & Robert, 2013).

The question, then, is whether and how the programme takes into consideration contextual issues in its organization and design, and whether it includes actions or interventions to address, transform or activate the multiple contextual factors at play in the different levels. Moreover, the assessment of the context should consider both positive and negative influences of other strategies, policies and programme.

Heterogeneity of subpopulations: Within a population, different subpopulations (e.g. as classified by place of residence, sex, socioeconomic status, etc.) have different needs and experiences in terms of health problems and health service access. Compared with the population as a whole, some subpopulations experience greater vulnerability or exposure to health risks and poorer access and outcomes in relation to health services. For example, gender shapes men's and women's roles and relations, their access to and control over resources, and their needs, including health needs. Likewise, populations living in rural areas often have poorer access to health and social services. The health programme must recognize and account for this heterogeneity in terms of the type, formulation and delivery of interventions and activities, as not doing so may directly or indirectly reinforce inequities.

Ultimately, realist evaluation assesses whether the programme interventions will produce the expected outcomes within the context and address heterogeneous needs and circumstances in order to work for the intended population (and the subpopulations). This requires unpacking the multiple contextual influences generating the underlying causes of inequities and subpopulation differences.

Programme interventions and mechanisms: The programme interventions produce mechanisms anticipated to produce changes aimed at improving the health of the target population. Frequently, health programmes address as causal mechanisms the set of genetic factors, specific exposures or behaviours ("lifestyle risk factors") associated with the progression of physiopathologic changes considered to be part of the "natural history" of disease. They often do not consider the social causes of these causes, which are found in the stratified social reality. However, abundant evidence confirms the existence of social gradients in the distribution of the causes of poor health, whose bases are social stratification mechanisms generating inequities in power, resources, prestige and discrimination (CSDH, 2008). These social differences affect the likelihood of health damaging or protective exposures, vulnerabilities and access to health and other services, which are the mechanisms of health inequities across the life course. (The mechanisms of inequities in relation to the programme will be examined in Step 5.)

The transformative potential of a programme to change the generative processes of the stratified social reality in which it is embedded is defined, according to Pawson and Tilley (2004), by the interplay of context, programme mechanisms and outcomes. The context can be seen as a vibrant mix of programme actions and other events within the system of social relations and structures that uniquely occur in a specific time and place, which activate, block or modify a chain of causal mechanisms, potentially leading to very different outcomes according to the dynamics at play. Thus, programme mechanisms encompass the reasoning and reactions of the agents, who seek to bring about change through the implementation of an intervention, interacting with the target population in a specific context.

Complexity of programmes: Public health programmes are complex, often made up of various interventions, encompassing several component mechanisms, and occurring in dynamic contexts, where social relations and structures and other interventions affect outcomes.

Unpacking this complexity to understand the essential mechanisms or functions of the programme and the varying forms it takes in different contexts is a challenging process, which the Innov8 methodology seeks to facilitate. This specific step is about uncovering and articulating the current reasoning on how and why the programme should work to produce the expected results. In the upcoming steps, the review team will examine whether and how this theory of the programme works or fails for different subpopulations. This testing allows the review team to uncover the processes generating inequities in relation to the programme, in order to reveal the "theory of inequities" operating in relation to the programme, which should be addressed in a redesign proposal. This will result in a revised programme theory, a theory of change that encompasses issues of equity, gender, human rights and social determinants of health.

Step 2 Additional reading and resources

Mkandawire T (2005). Targeting and Universalism in Poverty Reduction. United Nations Research Institute for Social Development. Social Policy and Development Programme Paper Number 23. Geneva: UNRISD. Available: http://www.unrisd. org/80256B3C005BCCF9/search/955FB8A594EE A0B0C12570FF00493EAA?OpenDocument (accessed 18 February 2016).

Pawson R, Sridharan S (2009). Theory-driven evaluation of public health programmes. In: Killoran A, Kelly M, eds. Evidence-based public health: Effectiveness and efficiency. Oxford: Oxford University Press: 43–61.

CASE STUDY EXAMPLE OF STEP 2 FROM A COUNTRY PROGRAMME APPLICATION

This example draws from the colorectal cancer screening programme of the Basque Government of Spain. In 2010–2011, a review team was constituted to conduct a programme review within the broader Spanish Government's training process to integrate social determinants of health and health equity into health strategies, programmes and activities at national, regional and local levels (as part of Spain's National Strategy on Health Equity). The programme diagram of the key stages of the screening programme and the programme theory developed by the review team are shown here as an illustrative example of outputs from Step 2.

Figure 2.2 Key stages of the screening programme for colorectal cancer of the Basque Government of Spain

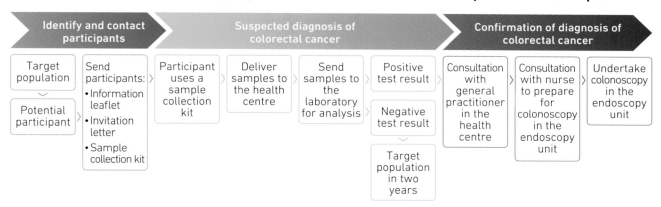

The programme theory of the screening programme for colorectal cancer

By sending a letter and information leaflet to all people aged 50 to 69 years living in the administrative area, inviting them to participate in the colorectal cancer screening programme, the programme assumes that they will receive, read and understand the letter; and expects that 60% of those contacted will be motivated to bring a stool sample to the health centre for faecal occult blood testing. This is facilitated by long opening hours and telephone question and advice call lines. In the case of a positive test result, the participant will be given a timeslot for consultation with a general practitioner, which it is assumed that they will keep, and once informed will accept to undergo a colonoscopy (including the preparations for it). Following a consultation with a general practitioner all participants have an appointment with a nurse in preparation for the colonoscopy appointment. The programme also expects that people who obtained a negative result in the first round (>92%), will continue participating in the programme when a letter is sent to them again two years after the first round, and they will again collect and submit a sample for faecal occult blood testing.

Sources: WHO, 2013; Ministry of Health, Social Services and Equality, Government of Spain, 2012; Merino et al, 2014; Portillo et al, 2015.

UNDERSTAND THE PROGRAMME THEORY
STEP 2

STEP 2 ACTIVITIES SUMMARY

The activities of Step 2 aim to guide the review team in uncovering the programme theory. The step focuses on the current programme (i.e. not on what the team aspires to do in the redesign phase).

Often a programme is highly complex, with multiple subprogrammes and interventions, which makes it difficult to review all of the different components.

Therefore, the review team may choose to prioritize some components of the programme for review. This decision should consider the potential impacts on equity, gender, human rights and social determinants of health.

Table 2.1 summarizes the activities that the review team will carry out to develop Step 2.

Table 2.1 Summary of activities to develop Step 2: Understand the programme theory

Questions	Tasks	Methods
Activity 1: Conceptualize the problem(s) or topic(s) to be addressed		
What is the problem to be addressed?	• Refine the statement of the problem ("problem space") the programme is designed to address, reviewing checklist question 2.	Review of programme documents and checklist findings Team discussion
Activity 2: Programme solution space – organize interventions, services or activities in key stages		
What does the programme specifically do to address the problem? Which activities are being implemented to produce progress on which outcomes?	• Review the programme activities and organize them in components or key stages that produce progress towards an outcome. • Classification of the interventions: downstream, midstream, upstream and universal versus selective or mixed.	Review of programme documents and checklist findings Team discussion
Activity 3: Build a diagram with the programme's key stages		
What are the key stages of the programme?	• Build a logic model diagram of the programme key stages (sequence of activities) linked to the outputs and outcomes.	Review of documents and checklist findings Team discussion
Activity 4: Write a summary of the programme theory		
What is the programme theory?	• Write a statement of the programme theory and, if necessary, adjust the diagram to better reflect the theory statement.	Review of documents and checklist findings Team discussion
Activity 5: How are equity, gender, human rights and social determinants considered in the programme?		
How does the programme take into account context and heterogeneity? Does the programme include action on social determinants, gender and human rights?	• Review whether the current programme theory explicitly considers context, heterogeneity and social determinants, gender and human rights issues. • If necessary, adjust the programme theory statement and programme diagram.	Review of documents and checklist findings Team discussion

STEP 2 ACTIVITY GUIDE

ACTIVITY 1

Conceptualize the problem(s) or topic(s) to be addressed

Understanding the programme theory begins with specifying **the problem or topic addressed by the programme,** which its objectives and lines of action seek to change. The problem space provides knowledge of what variables or systems of relationships are associated with the health outcome. Remember: outputs are different from outcomes. While outcomes describe the actual impact (the change that results), outputs simply describe the quantity of services provided (Taylor-Powell & Henert, 2008).

Sometimes when defining the problem to be addressed, health professionals simply describe implementation

problems related to health system functions, such as weak referral systems, or the inputs of the programme, i.e. human resources or budgetary constraints. But this is not the same as the health problem or topic affecting the population that the programme aims to act on. Table 2.2 shows three illustrative and hypothetical examples. The first focuses on an infectious disease programme, which aims to reduce mortality and sequelae associated with the infection. Programme interventions to achieve these objectives are primarily in the area of prevention; focusing on immunization. The second hypothetical example is for a non-transmissible chronic disease, hypertension, and the third is for adolescent sexual health.

Table 2.2 Examples of the problem and solution spaces of different types of health programmes

Programme	Measles	Non-communicable disease	Adolescent sexual health
PROBLEM SPACE			
Problem to be addressed	Mortality and morbidity by measles	Control of hypertension, diabetes, smoking, obesity and other conditions related to cardiovascular morbidity and mortality	Healthy sexuality and teenage pregnancy and sexually transmitted infections (STIs)
SOLUTION SPACE			
Impact	Reduce the mortality and eliminate cases of measles	Reduce the incidence of hypertension and other conditions, cardiovascular complications and disabilities	Reduce adolescent fertility rates and STI incidence in adolescents
Interventions or activities (outputs)	Vaccines for measles, education for communities, others	Regulation of salt content, education, screening and control activities	Health education, counselling and free contraceptives
Outcome*	Coverage of vaccine	Grams of sodium consumed, percentage screened and control of hypertension	Lower levels of unmet need for contraception, higher levels of knowledge
Inputs	Human resources to vaccinate, vaccines, transport, etc.	Human resources for enforcement, screening and control activities, medicine	Trained teachers and health personnel, infrastructure, contraceptives, etc.

* In some frameworks coverage is considered to be an output measure, while outcome is used for results that reflect expected changes in the target population rather than system productivity. Impact usually refers to longer term results, such as reduction in mortality.

UNDERSTAND THE PROGRAMME THEORY
STEP 2

A more comprehensive approach to the definition of the problem considers the need to address health inequities, i.e. the programme sets inequity as a problem in and of itself. Other broader approaches might look at results beyond the absence of disease or disability, i.e. such as establishing as programme concerns, the quality of life of people with measles or of amputees and those blinded due to diabetes complications, with specific programme actions to address these situations. See the examples in Table 2.3.

Table 2.3 The problem and solution space of equity-oriented health programmes

Programme	Measles	Non-communicable disease	Adolescent sexual health
Problem that includes inequity	Differential access to vaccination, exposure to virus, vulnerabilities and consequences of infection by sex, low socioeconomic position, migrant status, ethnic minority status	Differential effective coverage for treatment of hypertension and its potential health consequences (e.g., by sex due to gender-related barriers, by geography due to transport barriers, by income due to financial barriers)	Differences in availability, accessibility, acceptability of adolescent friendly health services and contraception by sex, age and neighbourhood, and increased risky sexual behaviour in adolescents from marginal families or out-of-school adolescents
Selected interventions or activities	Additional or differential interventions for low income communities and migrant families, gender-sensitive and culturally appropriate information, education and communication (IEC)	Additional or differential interventions for low income communities including to address gender norms, roles and relations that are harmful to health	Additional or differential interventions for low income communities and school dropouts, including that consider and aim to transform harmful gender norms, roles and relations
Equity impact	Reduce gaps of mortality and morbidity caused by measles by sex, income levels, migrant and non-migrant and between minority and majority ethnic groups	Reduce gaps in the incidence of complications of uncontrolled hypertension by sex and between income and education levels	Reduce differential teen pregnancies by sex, household deprivation and by in-school/out-of-school status

1. **After reflecting on the above considerations, the review team should write a summary of the problem to be addressed by the programme in no more than one paragraph.**

Example 2.1 shows a problem statement for a child health programme for a hypothetical country context.

Example 2.1 **Hypothetical example of a problem statement**

Children's health programme (0–9 years)

The problem addressed by the programme is as follows: congenital and perinatal conditions and other childhood diseases that are not prevented or diagnosed and treated in a timely and satisfactory way will lead to increased risks of disability and infant and child mortality. The lack of knowledge by parents or caregivers about nutrition and proper care, including immunization and stimulation, at different ages, produces illness and stunts development.

It should be noted that the programme does not explicitly consider that health equity issues are part of the problem, so the interventions are not intended to modify the collective social conditions that explain, in large measure, childhood exposures, vulnerabilities and health consequences.

ACTIVITY 2

Programme solution space – organize interventions, services or activities in key stages

The programme's solution space, i.e. the programme activities or interventions designed to address and influence the defined problem, are examined in this activity.

2.a. Review the main interventions, services or activities carried out in the programme and the relationship of these activities with the expected outcomes and longer term impact.

In checklist question 6, the review team listed the main programme interventions, services or activities and classified them as to whether they were directed at individuals or populations.

In this first task, the review team should examine this list and group the interventions or activities into the key stages of the programme related to a programme outcome(s).

Box 2.3 **Definition: key stage**

A key stage consists of a set of programme activities that are logically related to produce progress towards an outcome and impact. A key stage or a set of key stages may comprise an intervention. For example, screening may be an intervention, which encompasses the following activities: community outreach, distribution of information pamphlets, detection examinations, counselling, risk factor control and follow up, which may be broken down into various key stages with specific outputs and outcomes.

The overall programme outcome associated with the group of key stages related to screening is prevention of disease events through risk factor detection and control, but each key stage also has a more immediate outcome. If during screening, the presence of disease is detected, another programme intervention may be treatment of the disease to reduce morbidity, disability or mortality. In sum, more than one key stage may be associated with an outcome and a key stage may contribute to more than one outcome.

The following table may be useful for organizing the programme activities into key stages.

Key stage	Activities that are part of the key stage	Outcome(s) the key stage contributes to

2.b. Classify the main programme interventions using the following table.

A programme´s interventions work at different levels – downstream, midstream and upstream – depending on whether they focus more directly on curative health services, behaviours or wider determinants. Using the following table the team will first identify whether the intervention is downstream, midstream or upstream. Then, looking at the intervention programme coverage may be conceived of as an entitlement for the whole population, selectively directed to a certain targeted subpopulation or a combination of these approaches (called "mixed" coverage). In the table, each intervention should be placed in the appropriate row and column that describes its level of action and type of coverage. Completing this classification contributes to a better understanding of the intervention mechanisms or assumptions.

Complete the table by classifying the main programme interventions Type of coverage → Type of intervention ↓	Universal coverage (provided to the whole population)	Selective or targeted coverage (allocated on a selective basis according to a defined need or means testing)	Mixed coverage (combination of universal and selective)
Interventions to ensure access to health or social services or to curative care or secondary prevention (downstream)			
Interventions to influence behaviours and lifestyles (midstream)			
Interventions to influence living and working conditions (midstream)			
Interventions that seek to modify the broader context and/or the social stratification (upstream)			

Type of intervention by level of action:

- **Downstream** interventions aimed at addressing the **consequences generated by the problem**. For example: interventions to ensure access to curative care or secondary prevention actions (e.g. early detection of a health condition) or access to other social services.

- **Midstream** interventions that seek to **reduce the magnitude of exposures** or provide support to **address the greater vulnerability.** For example: interventions to influence behaviours and lifestyles; or interventions to influence living and working conditions.

- **Upstream** interventions that seek to modify the **broader context and/or social stratification**, i.e. tackle the inequitable distribution of power, money and resources (CSDH, 2008), that leads to certain subpopulations having higher exposure and vulnerability.

Type of coverage the programme is designed to provide:

- In programmes, **universal coverage** means intervention coverage or access is provided to the whole population of a country (e.g. all newborns are eligible for newborn care, all adolescents eligible for adolescent health services, all persons who have suffered a stroke are eligible for the appropriate

secondary prevention). These interventions are designed to benefit all people, regardless of their personal, social and economic characteristics (Raczynski, 1995).

- **Selective (targeted) coverage** is an intervention allocated on a selective basis, usually determined by a definition of need (for example, assessed by means testing of income).

- **Mixed coverage** is where the intervention coverage or access is a combination of universal and selective coverage, where the selectivity is used as an instrument to enforce or strengthen universalism. This has been referred to as "targeting within universalism", whereby the additional benefits are targeted to priority or high-need subpopulations (e.g. the lowest income group) in the context of a universal policy (Mkandawire, 2005).

If the programme includes selective coverage for a specific subpopulation, it may have an equity- or gender-specific aim. If the approach to coverage is mixed, it most likely has an objective for the whole target population as well as an equity- and/or gender-specific objective to ensure that no one "falls through the cracks"; i.e. certain subpopulations receive (more/adapted) services in accordance with their greater or specific needs and more adverse circumstances (progressive universalism).

ACTIVITY 3

Build a diagram with the programme's key stages

In Activity 2 of this step, the review team identified the set of activities that comprise the key stages of the programme. In Activity 3, these activities are illustrated in a diagram that represents an overview of the programme, showing the sequences of activities with arrows connecting the relationships between them that combine to produce the changes that lead to the programme outcomes. This is called a **logic model**, and will be referred to throughout the coming steps as the "programme diagram".

Multiple logic models might be necessary to depict a broad, complex programme. In this case, a global model may illustrate the overall programme while more specific logic models depict different levels, components or stages within the global programme. These constitute "families of logic models" or "nested logic models" (Taylor-Powell & Henert, 2008). As stated in the University of Wisconsin's teaching guidance on developing a logic model: "A single image that displays the programme theory is often the most difficult part of developing and using a logic model" (Taylor-Powell & Henert, 2008).

UNDERSTAND THE PROGRAMME THEORY
STEP 2

3.a. The review team can start by sequencing the set of programme key stages to show the flow and the linkages between the key stages and the programme results (outputs and outcomes). This provides an initial overview of the programme.

Initial diagram of the key stages of the programme

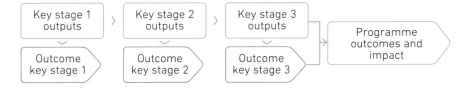

3.b. Enrich the initial diagram by developing logic models for key stages.

The above diagram can be made more explicative by unpacking the key stages with specific logic models for each one, which displays the connections between inputs (which may be specific or common to more than one key stage), the flow of outputs (activities and the people reached) and how these combine to produce the expected outcomes and impacts (see the definitions in Box 2.4). Depending on the complexity

of the programme, the number of key stages and the activities contained, this may result in a family of logic models. Alternatively, the team may choose to draw some of the key stages or only one. It is important to keep in mind that the diagram should provide an overview of the current programme (and not the changes that the review team wants to include in a redesign).

Enriched diagram of the key stages, including for each key stage

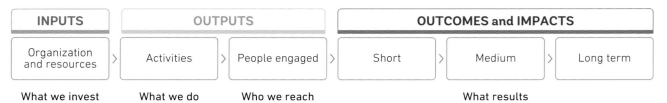

Box 2.4 Definitions: inputs, outputs, outcomes and impacts

Inputs: The resources that go into the programme and how they are organized for service delivery, including: staff (type), facilities, money, materials, equipment and volunteer time (what is invested).

Outputs: The goods, services or other activities delivered by the programme and who they reach. Who is reached is not the same as the target population. For example, a key stage of an adolescent health programme may be training of health staff and teachers in techniques to engage adolescents; who is reached are the health staff/teachers. The programme outputs are often described in terms of quantitative productivity and

coverage indicators (what the programme does and who it reaches).

Outcomes and impacts: The results or changes the programme is expected to achieve may be expressed in a continuum: usually target population service coverage indicators (outputs in some models and immediate outcomes in others) are associated with outcomes. Outcomes can be immediate or short term, intermediate, final or long term. Impact typically refers to changes in morbidity and mortality that have been influenced (acknowledging issues of attribution) by the coverage rates of the population with a set of services.

Sources: Drawing from WHO's results chain, WHO, 2014; Taylor-Powell & Henert, 2008.

In a complex, multilevel and multi-component programme, each model might depict the various programmatic components, goals, sites or target populations. Each of these "sub-models" and their expected outcomes link to the overall logic model to ensure that programmatic outcomes are achieved.

The review team may wish to develop **multilevel programme** nested logic models. For example,

a tobacco control programme may include macro (national) interventions such as a framework law prohibiting smoking in public places, advertising and restricting sales; in addition to institutional activities, such as enforcement and control activities; and at the community level, include youth prevention activities, environmental monitoring and smoking cessation activities. These multiple levels can be depicted with a series of nested models (Figure 2.3).

Figure 2.3 **A multilevel programme nested logic model**

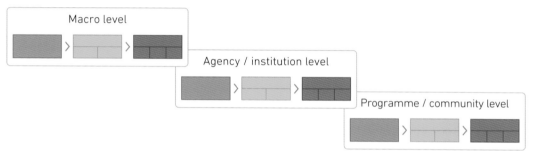

Source: Adapted from Taylor-Powell & Henert, 2008.

The macro level displays a global picture of a comprehensive national tobacco control strategy with several major programmes. These may include marketing prohibition and counter-marketing programmes, community programmes, a school programme and a chronic disease programme. Each of these can be described with its own logic model. The government agency responsible for tobacco control may also have several components, such as legislation and research, enforcement and evaluation and monitoring. At the community level the programmes engage directly with the population with promotion, prevention and treatment activities.

In this type of complex, multifaceted initiative at every level several models would detail the various programmatic components, goals, sites or target populations. Each of these "sub-models" and their expected outcomes links to the overall logic model to ensure that programmatic outcomes are achieved. For example, for a community-wide tobacco control programme, one "programme" logic model might provide the big picture of the total programme and then separate, "sub" logic models indicate the specific programme or components (Figure 2.4).

Figure 2.4 **Community tobacco control programme – three-year plan**

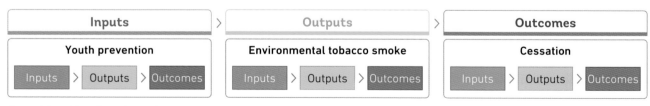

Source: Adapted from Taylor-Powell & Henert, 2008.

Specifically, the youth prevention programme might be displayed as follows (Figure 2.5).

Figure 2.5 Youth tobacco prevention programme

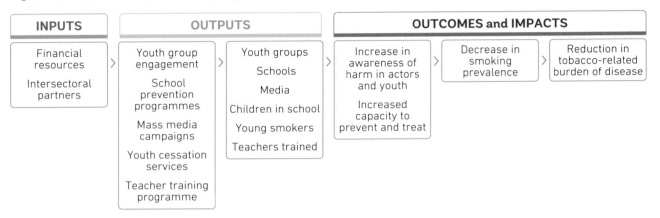

Source: Adapted from Taylor-Powell & Henert, 2008; Handout:34.

Remember, the logic model diagram is a "model" that displays the proposed causal connections between the inputs, outputs and outcomes of the programme, but it is not reality. However, even simple models are very useful for learning and innovation because they help clarify the expected pathways, uncover the underlying assumptions, test the linkages and orient policy-makers.

Some tips for developing the logic model:

- Use cards that can be pinned or taped to a board or wall and easily rearranged.

- Write one idea about inputs, outputs, outcomes and impacts on each card.

- Start by displaying the overall programme (all the key stages identified in Activity 2). Then decide if sub-models should be detailed (see the background reading for examples).

- It might be easier to brainstorm in groups of two or three then show the results to the rest of the team.

- Take a snapshot of the final product and then draw it using PowerPoint.

ACTIVITY 4

Write a summary of the programme theory

The summary statement of the programme theory explains why a programme is expected to work to change the problem for the target population. Whereas the diagram or logic model developed in the previous Activity 3 is a descriptive display of the linkages between inputs, outputs, outcomes and impact, which in part illustrates the theory. In this activity the review team will articulate a summary statement of the programme theory that explains how and why a programme is supposed to work. It provides a logical and reasonable description of why the programme activities should lead to the intended results or benefits. Programme theories can often be captured in a series of "if-then" statements – **if** something is done with or for the programme participants, **then** something should change.

To develop a programme theory, the review team should consider the following questions for the key programme stages. However, the review team does not need to develop a theory for everything in the programme; they should focus on the main services provided, i.e. the ones most central in obtaining positive results.

- **If** the activity is provided, **then** what – realistically – should be the result for the population?

- Why do you believe the activity will lead to this result? In other words, what is your assumption about how this kind of change occurs and how the target population will respond when they engage in this activity?

- What evidence do you have that the activity will lead to this result (such as previous results from your own or other programmes, published research or consistent feedback from participants)? Between the **if** and the **then** there should be some solid or some well-established connection supporting the idea that the service package will accomplish the programme goals.

4.a. After reflecting on these questions, write a summary of the programme theory in no more than three paragraphs.

For an example of the programme theory, please see the Case Study in this chapter. An additional example of the programme theory statement from a hypothetical children's health programme, based on different country experiences, follows.

Example 2.2 Hypothetical example of a programme theory statement

Children's health programme (0–9 years)
(continued from Example 2.1)

Programme theory: The programme is universal and includes preventive and curative services – including neonatal examination, regular check-ups, timely diagnosis, treatment and rehabilitation. It is assumed that these services will be available in all health facilities, and will be accessible for all. As such, all parents and caregivers bring their children to the health centre to receive these benefits. If the services were received, it was assumed that children would attain their maximum development, be diagnosed early and receive adequate treatment to recover health and avoid disability and mortality and have a good quality of life.

Reflective note: In articulating this programme theory, the review team became aware of the presence of health inequities in the child population, for example differences in infant mortality by level of maternal education. They recognized that the programme had not considered equity issues as part of the problem and did not have activities to reach children who might not be accessing it. Nor were there interventions aimed at families living in deprivation or with poor parenting skills. The review team began to think about whether what works to improve health at aggregate/country average level will have the same utility in reducing health inequities.

UNDERSTAND THE PROGRAMME THEORY
STEP 2

4.b. After completing the programme theory, the review team may want to incorporate into the logic model diagram they developed in the previous activity the assumptions about why the programme activities will produce the expected outcomes.

Box 2.5 Assumptions

Assumptions underlie much of what we do in programmes, including the beliefs we have about: how we think the programme will work, our ideas about the problem, how the participants learn and behave, their motivations, the external environment, the knowledge base, and the internal environment. For example, it might be assumed that: community coalitions are an effective strategy for addressing community problems; our partners

will participate actively in programme delivery; the funding will be adequate and available when needed; the target population will want to learn and change their behaviours.

Faulty assumptions are often the reason for poor results. It is often these underlying assumptions that hinder success or produce less-than-expected results. One benefit of the logical modelling is that it helps us make our assumption explicit.

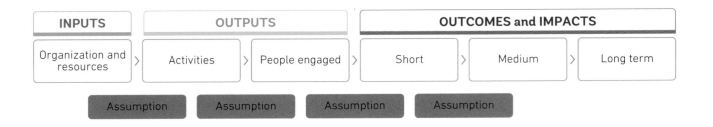

INPUTS	OUTPUTS		OUTCOMES and IMPACTS		
Organization and resources	Activities	People engaged	Short	Medium	Long term

Assumption   Assumption   Assumption   Assumption

ACTIVITY 5

How are equity, gender, human rights and social determinants considered in the programme?

The review team is now in a position to examine if and how the programme addresses issues related to equity, gender, human rights and social determinants.

It is not enough to have indicators or goals with an equity, gender or human rights focus (e.g. disaggregated by sex, urban/rural or other stratifier).

The question is whether the programme includes mechanisms (i.e. interventions and activities) aimed at reducing inequities and addressing issues related to social determinants, gender and human rights, and if so, what these entail. This requires examining in greater depth how the programme theory conceptualizes and addresses these issues.

5.a. In the formulation of the programme, is context as a central aspect included in the development of the programme?

As stated in the background reading at the start of this step, the **contexts** are contingent conditions that may alter the relationship between the programme and outcomes. The context may refer to national

policies, gender and community norms, institutional structures and cultural systems. Part of the context is the co-existence of other strategies, policies and programmes, as well as the overarching functionality of levels of the health system. These can influence the programme in synergistic or detrimental ways.

Please consider how the programme has identified actions or interventions to address these contexts, including the context of men's and/or women's lives and their different health needs, or how these contexts are considered in the programme organization. Include your answer in the table that follows 5.f.

5.b. In the formulation of the programme, is the heterogeneity of the target population (subpopulations) recognized and considered in programme interventions and actions?

That is, does it recognize different needs, circumstances, and, therefore, different interventions or actions? Will the programme work differently for different subpopulations, territories or individuals?

What actions are taken to prevent or address these differences? Include your answer in the table that follows 5.f.

5.c. In the formulation of the programme, is its impact on health equity explicitly defined?

Does the proposal address how health inequities are being generated in the problem or topic being addressed, the origin of health inequities and the impact of the programme on these health inequities?

As noted earlier, it is not enough to have an indicator or explicit goal on equity. Include your answer in the table that follows 5.f.

5.d. How are gender roles, norms and relations considered by the programme´s interventions and activities?

Are the different needs and experiences of men and women (which are shaped by gender roles, norms and relations) considered? Are men's and women's capacity to benefit from the programme considered? Do interventions and activities include ways to identify or address gender norms, roles and relations that are harmful for health? Do they consider how gender norms, roles and relations affect access to and control over resources? Does addressing gender inequality require specific activities for women or men of a particular group? Do programmatic materials or interventions reinforce gender-based stereotypes? Are programme delivery sites in places that both women and men can access? Include your answer in the table that follows 5.f.

5.e. Does the programme formulation reflect human rights principles such as equality and non-discrimination, participation and accountability? Include your answer in the following table.

How does the programme address these human rights principles such as equality and non-discrimination, participation and accountability?

5.f. The key question the review team is trying to answer is: **Are there any interventions or courses of action in the programme actually aimed at achieving greater equity in health, addressing social determinants and/or acting on gender and human rights?**

UNDERSTAND THE PROGRAMME THEORY
STEP 2

Use the following table to summarize the discussion on the previous questions.

Checking the programme theory	Yes/ no	How is this aspect included/considered?
Does it include actions to address **social determinants**? Which determinants?		
Does it include the **context as a central aspect** in the development of programme? Is the context considered in defining the interventions of the programme?		
Is the **heterogeneity of the population** (or specific needs of different subpopulations) recognized and taken into consideration in the programme interventions (i.e. their design, content and intensity)?		
Are gender norms, roles and relations accounted for by the programme?		
Does the programme's formulation apply the principles of a human rights-based approach?		
Is the **impact on health equity** explicitly defined?		

The following hypothetical example draws from different country contexts on reflections on equity, gender, human rights and social determinants of health that emerged after responding to the above questions.

Example 2.3 **Hypothetical example**

Children's health programme (0–9 years)
(continued from Examples 2.1 and 2.2)

To contribute to equity in health is not currently an explicit goal of the programme. The children's health programme does not take into account that children of different population groups have different needs and circumstances, such as children in vulnerable living conditions and including differential needs of boys and girls, and does not have differentiated services. Therefore, the programme does not recognize, in practice, the heterogeneity of subpopulations.

The programme defines as risk groups those with biological vulnerability. It does consider the most vulnerable social groups to be families with an unemployed head of household and teenage mothers. The programme design does not identify and target the most vulnerable subgroups and it does not define specific intervention strategies for these groups in each key stage of the programme.

The programme does not account for gender norms, roles and relations. For example, it does not consider gender-based differentials for boy and girl children with regards to exposure, household-level investment in nutrition, care and education, access to and use of health services and social impact of ill-health. In addition the programme does not acknowledge the potential role of men as active caretakers or incorporate actions to actively engage male caretakers.

While it defines that actions should focus or concentrate on the most vulnerable groups, the actions offered to these groups are the same as for the entire population. This means that although the contexts are considered in formulating the programme, this doesn't translate into different activities and implementation modalities of the programme for these groups.

Finally, the review team discussion identified that there are two groups of actions with limited development or that are virtually absent from the children's programme:

1. Actions proposed to other sectors of the state – public policies aimed at **reducing specific exposure to health damaging factors** suffered by families and children in disadvantaged positions (e.g. improving housing conditions, work, security, public spaces, restricting sales of tobacco and alcohol, food security, elimination of environmental pollutants, etc.).

2. Actions aimed at families and caregivers of children – aimed at **reducing the vulnerability of disadvantaged families and individuals**. For children and their families, these actions are those that constitute the health component (complementary and integrated with education and social security actions) of the social protection system for children. For example, due to gender roles, women and girls often bear an undue portion of the burden of home-based care-giving responsibilities, in addition to their other activities. Evidence also suggests that male involvement can improve physical and psychosocial child health outcomes. Part of these actions also include services developed by other health programmes, including family planning, activities to address gender-based violence, for breast feeding in the workplace, and for the cessation of tobacco alcohol and drugs consumption, among others.

After concluding this discussion, if necessary, the review team might want to revise the programme diagram and statement of the programme theory.

But remember at this stage, any changes should continue to reflect the programme as it is now (prior to revision and redesign).

UNDERSTAND THE PROGRAMME THEORY
STEP 2

STEP 2 OUTPUTS

Congratulations, the review team has completed the analysis for Step 2!

The review team should **summarize the outputs of Step 2 in a short report (approximately two to five pages)**, while this analysis is fresh in your minds. The output summary should clearly and succinctly capture the main findings and decisions of the review team across the activities in this step. You will be using this output across the steps, steadily building on it.

The output summary for Step 2 should cover the following components:

• A brief statement of the programme theory that explains the logical flow of the activities and how these will lead to the intended results, including any assumptions about how these activities should work to produce the expected outputs and outcomes.

• The diagram with programme key stages (that shows the sequence of activities of the programme key stages linked to the outputs and outcomes).

• A description of whether and how the current programme theory explicitly considers context, heterogeneity and equity, gender, human rights and social determinants of health issues.

REFERENCES

CSDH (2008). Closing the gap in a generation: Health equity through action on the social determinants of health. Final Report of the Commission on Social Determinants of Health. Geneva: World Health Organization. Available: http://whqlibdoc. who.int/publications/2008/9789241563703_eng.pdf (accessed 22 February 2016).

de Souza DE (2013). Elaborating the Context-Mechanism-Outcome configuration (CMOc) in realist evaluation: A critical realist perspective. Evaluation. 2013;19:141–54.

Fulop N, Robert G (2013). Context for successful quality improvement. London: The Health Foundation.

Lacouture A, Breton E, Guichard A, Ridde V (2015). The concept of mechanism from a realist approach: a scoping review to facilitate its operationalization in public health program evaluation. Implementation Science. 2015;10(1):153. Available: http://www.implementationscience.com/content/10/1/153 (accessed 18 February 2016).

Merino B, Campos P, Gil Luciano A (2014). Presentation: Overview of the review and redesign process. WHO meeting in Alicante, Spain. June 2014.

Ministry of Health, Social Services and Equality, Government of Spain (2012). Methodological guide to integrate equity into health strategies, programmes and activities. Version 1. Madrid. Available: http://www.msssi.gob.es/profesionales/saludPublica/prevPromocion/promocion/desigualdadSalud/jornadaPresent_Guia2012/docs/Methodological_Guide_Equity_SPAs.pdf (accessed 17 February 2016).

Mkandawire T (2005). Targeting and Universalism in Poverty Reduction. United Nations Research Institute for Social Development. Social Policy and Development Programme Paper Number 23. Geneva: UNRISD. Available: http://www.unrisd.org/80256B3C005BCCF9/search/955FB8A594EEA0B0C12570FF00493EAA?OpenDocument (accessed 18 February 2016).

Pawson R, Sridharan S (2009). Theory-driven evaluation of public health programmes. In: Killoran A, Kelly M, eds. Evidence-based public health: Effectiveness and efficiency. Oxford: Oxford University Press: 43–61.

Pawson R, Tilley N (1997). Realistic evaluation. London: Sage.

Pawson R, Tilley N (2004). Realist evaluation. London: British Cabinet Office. Available: http://www.communitymatters.com.au/RE_chapter.pdf (accessed 18 February 2016).

Portillo I, Idigoras I, Bilbao I, Hurtado JL, Urrejola M, Calvo B, Mentxaka A, Hurtado JK (2015). Programa de cribado de cáncer colorectal de euskadi. Centro Coordinador del Programa de Cribado, Subdirección de Asistencia Sanitaria, Dirección General de Osakidetza, Bilbao. Available: http://www.osakidetza.euskadi. eus/contenidos/informacion/deteccion_cancer/es_cancer/ adjuntos/programa.pdf (accessed 17 February 2016).

Raczynski D (1995). Focalización de programas sociales. Lecciones de la experiencia Chilena. In: Pizarro C et al, eds. Políticas económicas y sociales en el Chile democrático. Corporación de Investigaciones Económicas para Latinoamérica-United Nations Children's Fund, Santiago, Chile. [English version, 1996, Social and economic policies in Chile's transition to democracy.]

Rogers PJ (2000). Causal models in program theory evaluation. New Directions for Evaluation. 2000;87:47–55.

Sridharan S (2009). Ten steps to making evaluation matter. Presentation at Evaluation Workshop, Santiago, Ministry of Health, Chile. Sanjeev Sridharan, University of Toronto and Centre for Urban Health Research at St Michael's Hospital.

Sridharan S (2012). A Pocket Guide to Evaluating Health Equity Interventions – Some Questions for Reflection by Sanjeev Sridharan, Magic: Measuring & Managing Access Gaps in Care (blog entry). Available: http://www.longwoods.com/blog/a-pocket-guide-to-evaluating-health-equity-interventions-some-questions-for-reflection/ (accessed 18 February 2016).

Sridharan S, Gnich W, Moffat V, Bolton J, Harkins C, Hume M, Nakaima A, MacDougall I, Docherty P (2008). Independent evaluation of Have a Heart Paisley Phase 2. Evaluation of the Phase 2 primary prevention. Edinburgh: University of Edinburgh, Research Unit in Health, Behaviour and Change. Available: http:// www.healthscotland.com/uploads/documents/8266-Primary_ Prevention_HAHP2.pdf (accessed 28 February 2016).

Taylor-Powell E, Henert E (2008). Developing a logic model: Teaching and training guide. Madison, WI: University of Wisconsin-Extension Cooperative Extension, Program Development and Evaluation. Available: http://www.uwex. edu/ces/pdande/evaluation/evallogicmodel.html (accessed 18 February 2016).

WHO (2013). Integration of social determinants of health and equity into health strategies, programmes and activities: Health equity training process in Spain. Social Determinants of Health discussion paper 9. Geneva: World Health Organization. Available: http://apps.who.int/iris/ bitstream/10665/85689/1/9789241505567_eng.pdf (accessed 18 February 2016).

WHO (2014). Twelfth General Programme of Work 2014–2019. Geneva: World Health Organization.

Step3

Identify who is being left out by the programme

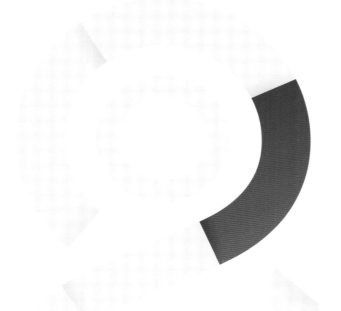

Overview

In Step 3, the review team examines who is being left behind by the programme. It entails analysing which subpopulations are really accessing, receiving interventions and obtaining the benefits at each key stage of the programme and – most importantly from an equity, gender and human rights perspective – which are not or do so to a lesser extent.

Step 3 considers each of the subpopulations that compose the programme´s target population, to analyse their different experiences with regard to programme processes, outputs and results. Programmes may "work" differently and have different outcomes for different subpopulations. This is also in relation to differences across the stages of a programme.

This examination of subpopulation differences serves to "test" the programme theory to see what is happening in practice. It tests its capacity to address the heterogeneous requirements of various subpopulations and access and benefiting by the most vulnerable groups in comparison to more privileged groups. In essence, Step 3 tests the programme theory's potential to contribute to health equity, gender equality and attainment of the right to health for all.

The four activities of Step 3 guide the review team towards:

1) Preliminarily assessing which subpopulations experience inequities in the programme;

2) Characterizing the subpopulations and their differential needs;

3) Testing the preliminary analysis using quantitative and qualitative information; and

4) Revising the programme diagram to indicate which subpopulations are not accessing or benefiting at each key stage, as well as identifying and prioritizing the subpopulation(s) of the programme for further analysis.

The analysis builds on the findings from the previous steps, as well as on other data sources identified by the review team.

The main outputs of Step 3 are an assessment of the differential heath needs and differences in programme access and coverage across the target population groups, leading to the prioritization of the subpopulation(s), which will be considered for further analysis in the review process.

Objectives of Step 3

> Identify and characterize relevant subpopulations of the programme's target population in terms of their socioeconomic position and social stratification mechanisms. Consider gender and its intersections with other stratification mechanisms.

> Apply quantitative and qualitative techniques to analyse subpopulation differences and relative disadvantages, and whether or not the relevant subpopulations are accessing and benefiting from each key stage of the programme.

> Identify and prioritize the subpopulations excluded or in situation of inequity in each key stage and the most critical key stages of the programme in terms of exclusion or inequities.

IDENTIFY WHO IS BEING LEFT OUT
BY THE PROGRAMME
STEP 3

BACKGROUND READING FOR STEP 3

Concepts and methods to identify, characterize and prioritize who does and does not benefit from the programme

The following reading aims to provide a basic orientation for thinking about who accesses and benefits from the programme and *who does not*, before the review team begins to complete the work for Step 3. The reading covers:

- Socioeconomic position and social stratification (including gender norms, roles and relations);
- Relevance of the "grounds of discrimination" (including by sex, race/ethnicity, etc.);

- Socioeconomic position, health need and demand for health services;
- Common approaches to measuring social differences; and
- Data sources and methods for measuring health inequalities.

Socioeconomic position and stratification

When considering the subpopulations who may or may not be benefiting from the health programme, it is useful to consider socioeconomic position as a starting point. People attain different positions in the social hierarchy according, mainly, to their social class, educational achievement, occupational status and income level.

Socioeconomic position refers to the social and economic factors that influence the positions individuals or groups hold within the structure of a society. It is a term that encompasses the various measures that reflect the position of individuals or groups in the social hierarchy.[1] It is understood as an aggregate concept that includes integrated measurement of access to and control over resources and prestige in society, linking these with social class. For examples, see Marx, Weber, Krieger, Williams and Moss (Krieger et al, 1997; Galobardes et al, 2006).

Two major variables used to operationalize socioeconomic position in monitoring health inequities are social stratification and social class. **Social stratification** refers to social systems that categorize or rank individuals or subpopulations in a hierarchy according to some attribute, resulting in structured social inequality. Income, years of education and type

of occupation are familiar examples of attributes used in this ranking process. Gender norms, roles and relations can also contribute to unequal power relations. These rankings or scales are known as simple **scales graduation**. **Social class** is defined by the ratio of ownership and control over the means of production, whether physical, financial or organizational. Social class is known as a **relational measure**, because changes in the social situation of one category necessarily impact on the other category or categories.

Measures of social stratification are important predictors of patterns of mortality and morbidity. There are two main entry points for measurement associated with socioeconomic position:

- **Resource-based measures** refer to material and social resources and assets, including income, wealth and educational credentials; terms used to describe inadequate resources include poverty and deprivation.

- **Prestige-based measures** refer to an individual ranking or status in the social hierarchy, typically evaluated in terms of the level in magnitude and quality of access and consumption of goods, services and knowledge. These measures include occupation, education and income, which relate to prestige in given contexts.

---

[1] A variety of other terms, such as social class, social stratum and social or socioeconomic status, are often used more or less interchangeably in the literature, despite their different theoretical bases.

As explained in the next section and illuminated in Figure 3.1, discrimination and social exclusion on the basis of gender and ethnicity both reflects and shapes one's position in the social hierarchy.

In addition, gender and ethnicity can interact with the other processes and characteristics which can lead to compounded disadvantage.

Figure 3.1 Mechanisms of distribution of power and their stratifiers

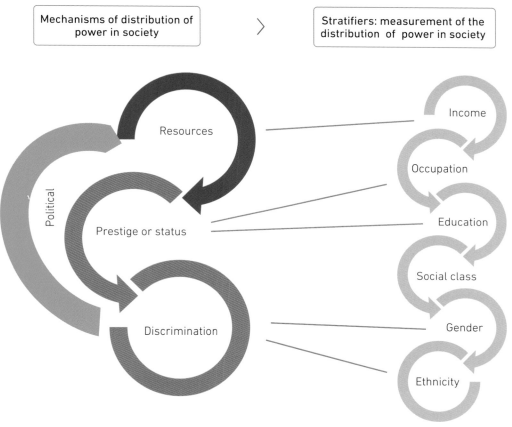

Source: Presentation of Innov8 elaborated by O Solar and P Frenz.

Relevance of the "grounds of discrimination"

Beyond resources and prestige, there are other measures that highlight important issues – such as discrimination – in relation to socioeconomic position that can be used for stratification. According to the United Nations Declaration of Human Rights (United Nations, 1948), the prohibited grounds of discrimination are identified as "race, colour, sex, language, religion, political or other opinion, national or social origin, property, birth or other status".

For example, across societies, discrimination based on sex or gender norms can affect health (WHO, 2011). An instance of this is when gender norms marginalize people whose gender identity and sexual orientation do not conform to the dominant ideals of a particular place or time. This can contribute to discrimination and, at times, violence.

The Convention on the Elimination of All Forms of Discrimination against Women (United Nations, 1979) addresses many of the ways in which discrimination can impact women's health, both directly and indirectly through discrimination's influence on socioeconomic position. Other conventions, such as the International Convention on the Elimination of All Forms of Racial Discrimination (United Nations, 1966), highlight additional forms of discrimination with implications for health.

Considerations on socioeconomic position, needs and effective coverage

Revisiting the conceptual framework of the social determinants of health, introduced in the section on *Introduction to applied concepts, principles and frameworks*, reinforces the understanding of the multiple pathways of socioeconomic position and health. In this framework, socioeconomic position influences an individual's material circumstances, behaviours and psychosocial factors, as well as their engagement with the health system. These, in turn, influence levels of equity in health and well-being experienced by an individual or subpopulations.

Figure 3.2 Conceptual framework of the social determinants of health, WHO

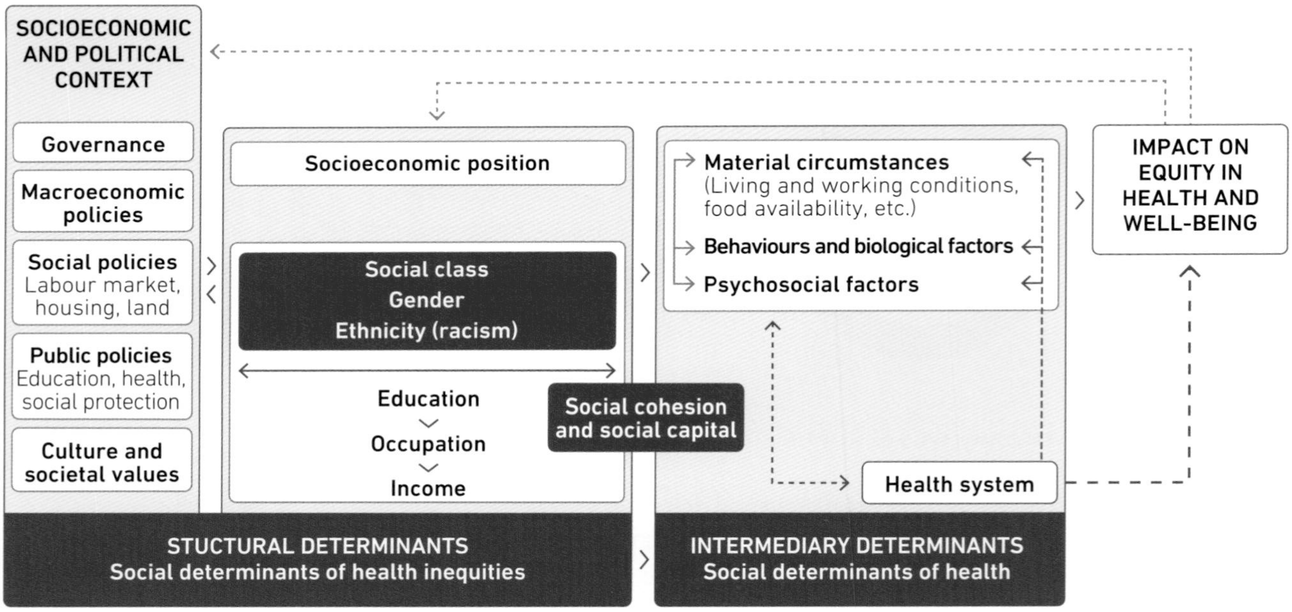

Source: Solar & Irwin, 2010.

Consistently, studies have demonstrated the existence of social gradients and differences in disease distribution in populations (CSDH, 2008). Yet, despite the greater health needs of individuals experiencing disadvantage – by income, education or precarious employment or by ethnicity, sex, gender, etc. – these subpopulations may not express demand or be able to access services or comply with treatments, resulting in lower levels of health service use in relation to their needs. Depending on the country context and the health programme, there may be situations of low use despite high need due to access barriers. So pervasive is this inequity in access it has been called the "inverse care law" (Tudor Hart, 1971). That said, Adler et al (1994) considered the role of access to care in explaining the socioeconomic position-related health gradient and concluded that access alone could not explain the gradient (pointing to the need to look at the role of determinants directly impacting health, as shown via the two solid arrows top right in Figure 3.2 that do not go through the health system box).

Some studies on this issue indicate that although gaps in access are larger between quintiles, people with lower income levels use more general practitioners and are hospitalized more than people of higher income, after taking into account the health need (Eckersley et al, 2001). At the same time, it has been confirmed that the use of specialist visits is reversed, because they are more often used by higher income people. The use of dental services is greater in people with higher incomes, a fact related to the exclusion of public funding in most countries (van Doorslaer et al, 2000; van Doorslaer, Koolman, Jones, 2004;

van Doorslaer et al, 2004). The evidence also suggests that screening and prevention programmes tend to benefit people from more affluent social classes more (De Spiegelaere et al, 1996; Alvarez-Dardet et al, 2001).

Thus, in interpreting programme outputs, it is important to consider differential needs (rates of disease or risk), and differential social circumstances (such as gender norms, roles and relations that may make women or men, or groups of women or men less likely to access and fully benefit from care despite potentially having greater or different needs). Equal use across social groups may in reality reflect inequities if use is not appropriate in quantity and quality to differential need. Table 3.1 may help the review team consider the current usage rates of subpopulations which have greater or different need. Time should be given to reflect on issues related to effective coverage of interventions (i.e. if the service the person can access is of sufficient quality).

Table 3.1 Different usage rates in relation to need

		NEED	
		HIGH	LOW
USE	HIGH	Appropriate access	Overuse
	LOW	Poor access	Appropriate access

Source: White, 1978.

Linked to the above, it is important to consider the conceptualization of the need existing in any given subpopulation and the expression of demand associated with such need. Different subpopulations within the target population – even if they have similar needs – may express this need differently due to their educational background, levels of health system literacy, experiences with discrimination, and/or prioritization of meeting basic needs related

to food and shelter, among other factors. Likewise, some subpopulations may express more need at certain health service usage points (for instance, in emergency rooms settings) that does not actually correlate with their level of needs for those specific services (CDC, 2013). Rather, this can be a reflection of challenges that the subpopulations face in accessing other parts of the system.

Common approaches to measuring stratification

Subpopulations and their socioeconomic position can be measured using different stratifiers, including those used to monitor health inequality. Reviewing these

indicators can help the review team characterize the subpopulations of the target population, who may be benefiting less or more from the programme.

There is no single best indicator suitable for all study aims and applicable at all time points in all settings. Each indicator measures different, often related, aspects of socioeconomic stratification and it is therefore often preferable to look at multiple aspects rather than only one. Some indicators may be more or less relevant to different health outcomes and at different stages in the life course. Examples across the life course include infancy, childhood, adolescent, adult, or, alternatively, time periods such as in the past year, five years, and so on. Relevant time periods depend on presumed exposures, causal pathways and associated etiologic periods. Socioeconomic position can also be measured meaningfully at three complementary levels: individual, household and neighbourhood. It is prudent to consistently look at differences between men and women, and girls and boys when considering other types of stratification, in order to see the potential gender/sex-related differences amongst subpopulations defined by different characteristics.

Some of the most frequently used stratifiers in monitoring health inequality include (WHO, 2013):

• Income or wealth;
• Place of residence (rural, urban, other);
• Race or ethnicity;
• Occupation (workers/employed, unemployed);
• Sex;
• Religion;
• Education;
• Socioeconomic status;
• Social class;
• Age; and
• Other characteristics particularly important for the programme and country context (e.g. migrant status, caste, gender identity and sexual orientation).

As described earlier, these and other stratifiers are used as proxy measures to measure the mechanisms for the distribution of resources, prestige or status, and discrimination in society, as illustrated in Figure 3.1. Therefore, due attention should also given to intersections between these characteristics. That is, reflecting how material disadvantage, low prestige and discrimination generated by social stratification mechanisms, converge to make some subpopulations particularly at risk of not benefiting from a programme (e.g. having low education *and* living in an urban informal settlement *and* being poor *and* being a woman). Area measures such as the Human Development Index or multidimensional poverty indexes, available in some countries by smaller geographical units, can also be relevant.

Data sources and methods for measuring health inequalities

For Step 3, the review team is asked to review and interpret available quantitative and qualitative data sources that give insights to subpopulation differences related to programme access, outputs and results.

Quantitative data sources: Useful to consider are population-based sources (censuses, vital registration systems and household surveys), institution-based sources (resource, service and individual records), and surveillance systems (WHO, 2013). Other important data sources include previous programme reviews and evaluations, studies from other population-based sources, as well as reviews of data accessible through articles in different search databases.

From these sources, important information can be drawn including:

• Process, output, results and impact indicators, including those used by the programme, which can be disaggregated (at least by sex and territory).

• Institute- or population-based data applicable for equity and gender analysis, for example by geographic unit like district and state, place of residence (rural/urban), sex, income, education and other relevant equity stratifiers appropriate for the national context.

• Information on subpopulations and coverage gaps, among others.

In some situations, there may be a lack of national data – across all key stages of the programme – or an inability to disaggregate by the stratifiers that the review team feels are most important. In this situation, it may be possible to review data disaggregated by the relevant stratifiers at a subnational or local level, drawing from smaller/localized data sources. If there is no disaggregated quantitative information at any level, the analysis could be done by geographic units, such as municipalities or county, selecting a group of localities that reflect differential rates of vulnerability, including social factors such as poverty and presence of subpopulations experiencing high levels of discrimination and social exclusion (e.g. ethnic minorities/tribal populations).

Table 3.2 provides a review of some simple epidemiological measures commonly used to analyse inequalities in health.

Table 3.2 Epidemiological measures commonly used to analyse inequalities in health

Measure	Calculation formula	Interpretation	Strengths
Percentage distribution of cases and population by social groups	Percentage of cases in each subpopulation (e.g. % of child deaths and % of births, according to maternal education groups).	Percentage of differences in coverage of services should consider differences in needs as well. If it is lower than expected according to the level of need, there is probably a situation of inequity.	Simple presentation of disproportions that reflect an uneven burden of health problems and health access.
Specific rates of social group	Number of cases in the social group divided by the population of the social group (e.g. infant mortality rate/ maternal education groups).	The specific rate of each social group represents the probability of the event (risk) of that social group.	Specific rates, especially using a graphic presentation, illustrate social gradients in health.
Ratio of observed cases and expected cases	Compares the ratio of observed cases in the social group with the expected cases.	The relationship of observed cases to expected cases is 1 if service use is equal to the group's needs. If it is <1 use is lower than expected.	Simple comparison of differences in observed and expected numbers of cases or people in the programme.
Absolute difference	Percentage coverage in low-income group subtracted from the percentage coverage in the high-income group.	The absolute difference measures the size of the differences. This should be compared with the absolute difference in need.	It is an indicator of the magnitude of the problem, reflecting its importance to public health.
Relative difference or ratio	Level of coverage in the best-off versus the worst-off.	The relative difference measures the magnitude of the effect of socioeconomic position in the measured phenomenon. If it is >1 or <1 a difference exists. Again, it should be contrasted with need.	It is considered a better indicator of the causal effect than the absolute difference.
Population attributable risk	Summary measure of gradient.	Shows possible improvements in health coverage by eliminating all socioeconomic differences.	Takes the size of groups into account.

Sources: Based on Mackenbach & Kunst, 1997; Galobardes et al, 2006; Jurges et al, 2008; elaborated from Ministerio de Salud, Chile, 2010; and revised according to WHO, 2013 and WHO, 2015.

IDENTIFY WHO IS BEING LEFT OUT BY THE PROGRAMME
STEP 3

Qualitative data sources: The value of qualitative data should not be underestimated, and can provide critical information on subpopulations being missed by the programme, their needs, access barriers and causes of inequities. If the programme has not collected qualitative data, sources that feature qualitative data may include, among others:

• Academic research and literature;

• Voices of male and female programme users from diverse communities;

• "Grey literature", such as reports from civil society and NGOs, National Human Rights Institutions, human rights treaty bodies and the media; and

• Reports from multilateral system partners.

Focus groups with the target population (and segments of it, including male and female users) and informant or in-depth interviews with local level providers and/or community members can provide essential insights into the reasons why some people may face challenges in accessing and benefiting from the programme, or any unintended consequences they experience as a result of using the programme (e.g. stigmatization). It is particularly important to look for data sources that cover both the perceptions from programme staff and health service providers (supply-side), as well as members of marginalized and disadvantaged communities (demand-side). Together, these sources provide critical insights about supply-side bottlenecks, perceptions of demand-side barriers and the potential causes of both that influence inequities.

Ultimately, the review team analysis in this manual considers **triangulating data from sources together with their own direct knowledge and experience to inform its reflections.** The review team´s perceptions and interpretations can be tested, verified or contrasted with these data sources and consultations with other people, especially local providers and managers.

Step 3 Additional reading and resources

Galobardes B, Shaw M, Lawlor DA, Lynch JW, Davey Smith G (2006). Indicators of socioeconomic position (part 1). Journal of Epidemiology and Community Health. 2006;60(1):7–12. doi: 10.1136/jech.2004.023531.

Krieger N (2001). A glossary for social epidemiology. Journal of Epidemiology and Community Health. 2001;55(10): pp.693–700. doi: 10.1136/jech.55.10.693.

Krieger N, Williams DR, Moss NE (1997). Measuring social class in US public health research: concepts, methodologies, and guidelines. Annual Review of Public Health. 1997;18:341–78. doi: 10.1146/annurev.publhealth.18.1.341.

UN CESCR (Committee on Economic, Social and Cultural Rights) (2009). General Comment No. 20: Non-Discrimination in Economic, Social and Cultural Rights, 02 July 2009, E/C.12/GC/20. Available: http://www.refworld.org/docid/4a60961f2.html (accessed 8 March 2016).

WHO (2014). Monitoring health inequality: An essential step for achieving health equity. Geneva: World Health Organization. Available: http://apps.who.int/iris/bitstream/10665/133849/1/WHO_FWC_GER_2014.1_eng.pdf?ua=1 (accessed 22 February 2016).

CASE STUDY EXAMPLE OF STEP 3 FROM A COUNTRY PROGRAMME APPLICATION

Chile´s cardiovascular health programme aims to detect and control major risk factors for cardiovascular disease in the adult population, 15 years and older, including hypertension, diabetes, dyslipidemia, overweight and tobacco, in primary care. In 2009–2010, the programme underwent a review and redesign process, within a broader review and redesign initiative that included five other programmes, to integrate health equity and social determinants of health perspectives in health programmes (as part of the Ministry of Health´s "13 steps towards equity" strategy).

To test the programme theory in terms of who was being left out, the review team (from the Ministry of Health and other sectors, including representatives from subnational levels) used available quantitative data from the 2003 National Health Survey in their analysis. This analysis revealed that only 60% of the adult population with hypertension was aware of their condition, a little more than a third were in treatment, and only 12% were normotensive (i.e. condition being successfully treated/managed) with important differences between men and women, as shown in Figure 3.3.

Figure 3.3 Rates of hypertension, National Health Survey, Chile, 2003

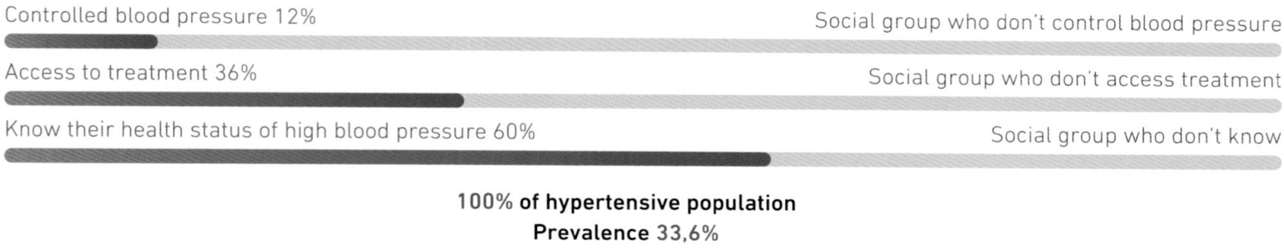

Controlled blood pressure 12% Social group who don't control blood pressure

Access to treatment 36% Social group who don't access treatment

Know their health status of high blood pressure 60% Social group who don't know

100% of hypertensive population
Prevalence 33,6%

Additional subnational information from the central Bío Bío Region (Figure 3.4) and the team's own knowledge and experience, verified through primary care programme registers, showed that the people accessing the cardiovascular health programme were mainly women, elderly and people who were not working.

Figure 3.4 Subnational level examples (Bío Bío Region cardiovascular health programme)

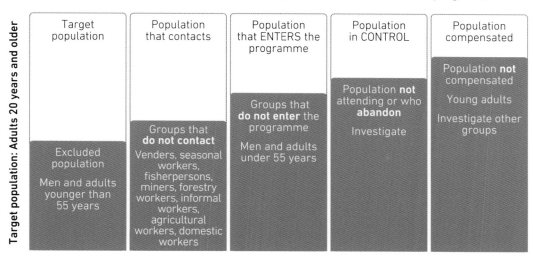

The critical key stages where people were being left behind are shown in the programme diagram (Figure 3.5).

Figure 3.5 Key stages where poorer working people, especially men, are left behind

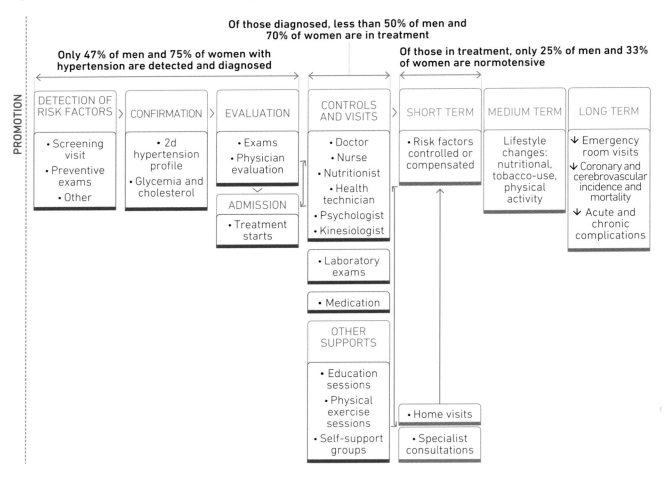

Sources: Ministerio de Salud, Chile, 2010; Solar, 2014; Vega, 2011.

The review team´s analysis concluded that the programme provided inadequate coverage, especially for men, in particular the working population aged between 45 and 60 years with social risk factors such as low education, unstable employment and low income, and residing in more disadvantaged districts. The subpopulation with these socioeconomic characteristics was considered to be the main excluded group from the programme, experiencing barriers to access for necessary health care.

STEP 3 ACTIVITIES SUMMARY

Table 3.3 contains the activities that the review team will develop to finalize Step 3. It also sets out the questions that orient the activities and the methods used.

Table 3.3 Summary of activities to develop Step 3: Identify who is being left out by the programme

Questions	Tasks	Methods
Activity 1: Preliminary assessment of the subpopulations who experience inequities in access or benefit less at each key stage of the programme		
For each key stage of the programme, which subpopulations might have more or less access or benefit?	• Preliminary analysis of subpopulation access/ benefits in key programme stages.	Team discussion
Activity 2: Characterize and describe the needs of the subpopulations		
Which subpopulations of the target population are important for the analysis? Characterize the subpopulations, using stratifiers.	• Characterize the subpopulations in the programme. • Identify differential needs of women and men from different subpopulations • Identify unintentional negative effects for any subpopulation. • Describe new or additional needs of this subpopulation that the programme does not address.	Review of programme documents and checklist findings Team discussion
Activity 3: Using quantitative and qualitative information to test the preliminary analysis of who is accessing and who is not, and which subpopulations have greater or different needs		
Do quantitative and qualitative data verify the preliminary assessment of the subpopulations who experience inequities?	• Identification of potential quantitative and qualitative data sources. • Verify and adjust the analysis using additional evidence and data.	Data source identification and compilation Review of evidence Consultation with informants Team discussion
Activity 4: Identify and prioritize the subpopulation(s) in situations of inequity		
Which subpopulation(s) and key stage(s) should be prioritized for further analysis?	• Revise the programme diagram to show which subpopulations are not accessing or benefiting at each key stage of the programme. • Indicate which subpopulation(s) are prioritized for further analysis.	Interpretation of findings Literature review Review team discussion

STEP 3 ACTIVITY GUIDE

The primary focus of the following exercises entails discussion and reflection by the review team, drawing on available information, about which subpopulations are accessing and benefiting at each key stage of the programme and which are not. The review team can draw from the checklist findings, programme documents, available quantitative and qualitative data sources, and their knowledge and experience.

ACTIVITY 1

Preliminary assessment of the subpopulations who experience inequities in access or benefit less at each key stage of the programme

The first activity of this Step 3 is to undertake a preliminary analysis, based on the knowledge and experience of the review team, of which subpopulations access and benefit and which do not at each key stage of the programme.

1. The review team should use the programme diagram and preliminary theory that they created in Step 2 to refer to the key stages of the programme.

With these in mind, they should consider how, for each key stage of the programme, some subpopulations might have more or less access or benefit. The review team is reminded to consider potential differentials based on sex or gender norms, roles and relations alongside other context-relevant stratifiers when defining the subpopulations. The review team may document their responses in the following table.

Key stage of the programme	Which subpopulation(s) access and benefit more	Which subpopulations do not access or benefit, or do so to a lesser extent

ACTIVITY 2

Characterize and describe the needs of the subpopulations

Based on the analysis about which subpopulations access and benefit or not at each key stage of the programme, in Activity 2, the review team should characterize the subpopulations of the programme's target population.

2. At this stage, the review team should review question 5 of the checklist and compare the subpopulations identified in this question with those identified in Activity 1 as accessing and benefiting more or to a lesser extent at the different programme stages. Then, in the left-hand column of the following table, they should put the complete list, listing also some descriptive characteristics including those that get at intersections. Again, consider potential differentials based on sex and/or gender norms, roles and relations and how these intersect with other social factors in this context. The review team should then complete the rest of the table. A hypothetical example of a sexual reproductive health programme is provided.

Subpopulation (brief description of characteristics)	In what way does the subpopulation have greater health needs? Why? What are they?	Does the programme have unintentional negative effects for this subpopulation?	Are there new or additional needs of this subpopulation that the programme does not address?
Example *(for a hypothetical sexual reproductive health programme):* Female labour migrants	**Example:** Female labour migrants may have limited access to health services due to lesser health system literacy and information access; gender, cultural and linguistic barriers; financial and administrative barriers; and informal working conditions with limited/no health-related benefits.	**Example:** The health system's and programme's exclusion of women in irregular status (without a working permit and residence visa) puts them at increased risk for not accessing timely services, and hence, experiencing exposure to risk factors, ill health and complications.	**Example:** The programme does not include integrated services to address gender-based violence, which is more prevalent among female labour migrants than among the general female population.

IDENTIFY WHO IS BEING LEFT OUT BY THE PROGRAMME
STEP 3

ACTIVITY 3

Using quantitative and qualitative information to test the preliminary analysis of who is accessing and who is not, and which subpopulations have greater or different needs

Activities 1 and 2 have resulted in a preliminary analysis about which subpopulations are accessing and benefiting and which are not, and which have greater or different needs. In Activity 3, the review team will test this preliminary analysis by reviewing existing available quantitative and qualitative data.

To complete this activity, the review team needs to have compiled available data sources, both quantitative and qualitative (see the background reading section). In relation to quantitative sources, it is necessary to consider the extent to which the data can be disaggregated for each subpopulation, using stratifiers (sex, income, education, occupation, race or ethnicity, etc.) and for different key stages of the programme.

In some country contexts and for some programmes, there may be a lack of quantitative data. If the problem is a lack of information at central level, it may be possible to find disaggregated data by subpopulation at the state/district or local level. In this case,

the review team should work with the local team to do the analysis or refer to existing local studies. If there is no disaggregated individual information, the analysis can be done by territory, such as municipalities or counties, selecting a group of localities that reflect different levels of vulnerability or differential rates of poverty or ethnicity.

Qualitative sources may provide information on specific subpopulations (and how different manifestations of disadvantage impact them) that is not available through quantitative means. If the review team decides to apply qualitative techniques such as focus groups and informant interviews, it should collect and systematize this information in relation to the subpopulations potentially being missed and stages of the programme. For example, the focus groups' participant profiles (from the demand-side) can reflect subpopulations who may not be accessing the programme. Informant interviews can be done with programme operators in low-income and/or rural remote areas.

3.a. Data verification of subpopulations who are accessing and those who are not.

Once the options for assessment of subpopulations and/or localities are decided, based on the available and collected information, the review team members should analyse the data to verify which subpopulations do not access and benefit or do so to

a lesser extent. The following table can assist with this (the review team can update the table done for Activity 1 by adding a new column and adjusting the contents as required).

Key stage of the programme	Verified subpopulations that do not access or benefit, or do so to a lesser extent	Verified subpopulations that access and benefit more	Verification done through which data sources (quantitative and qualitative)

3.b. Data verification of subpopulations with greater or different health needs.

For this exercise the review team may begin by referring to the content in the background reading section on differential needs and differential expression of those needs in relation to access and effective use of services. In particular, the team is encouraged to look at Table 3.1 regarding different usage rates in relation to need. Then, the review team should complete the following table, ticking how the evidence verifies types of differential needs, service usage and consequences of service use.

Subpopulations	Data sources			
	(list the data sources in each column that applies – if there are no data and sources, leave it blank)			
	Greater exposure and vulnerability to risk factors	Greater morbidity and mortality	Inappropriate use of services according to need	Social consequences (impoverishment, stigmatization, etc.) resulting from programme use

3.c. Calculation of relative ratio (RR) between subpopulations (optional exercise, according to data availability for subpopulations identified).

If sufficient quantitative data is available, the review team may try to measure the magnitude of the differences by calculating the relative ratio of the subpopulation with the lowest coverage in relation to the subpopulation with the best coverage or the average coverage of the target population.

Subpopulation	RR programme stage 1 (rate of subpopulation with lowest coverage/ rate of subpopulation with highest coverage)	RR programme stage 2 (rate of subpopulation with lowest coverage/ rate of subpopulation with highest coverage)	RR programme stage 3 (rate of subpopulation with lowest coverage/ rate of subpopulation with highest coverage)

ACTIVITY 4

Identify and prioritize the subpopulation(s) in situations of inequity

In the previous activities, the review team will have identified several subpopulations experiencing inequities in one of more of the programme's key stages. In this activity, the review team will map these subpopulations to the programme diagram and consider which subpopulations to prioritize for the continuation of the review.

4.a. Revised programme diagram featuring subpopulations being missed.

For this activity, the review team may go back to the programme diagram they developed in Step 2 and indicate in it which subpopulations are not accessing or benefiting at each key stage of the programme.

Who is left behind at each key stage of the programme

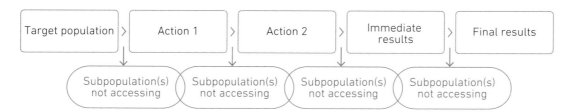

4.b. Prioritization of the subpopulation(s) for further analysis.

The next task is to consider which subpopulation(s) get prioritized for the continuation of the review. If the review team has the time and capacity, each of these subpopulations and key stages could be analysed in the following steps to build a comprehensive picture of inequities in relation to the programme. Given time or resource constraints, however, this may not be feasible.

In that case, the review team needs to prioritize the subpopulations that will be further analysed in subsequent steps and ultimately considered in the programme redesign. The review team needs to be able to justify *why* it has prioritized particular subpopulations. Table 3.4 describes commonly used criteria for prioritization that the review team may want to consider in making their decision. The review team may also want to further consider criteria in relation to gender mainstreaming in health programmes (WHO, 2011).

Table 3.4 Example criteria for prioritization

Criteria to identify priority problems (programmes)	Criteria to identify priority subpopulations	Criteria to prioritize interventions
Conceptualization (promotion, prevention, curative – upstream, downstream determinants)	Epidemiologic (magnitude, frequency)	Health equity impact
Impact (health, social)	Vulnerability (risk)	Effectiveness
Magnitude	Disadvantaged subpopulations (by sex, ethnicity, social class, etc.)	Expertise
Urgency	Social preference	Feasibility
Public and political connotations		Ease in implementation
Availability of solutions		Legal considerations
Cost of acting/not acting		System impacts
Responsibility		Return on investment
Considers gender norms, roles and relations for women and men and how they can affect access to and control over resources		Considers gender norms, roles and relations for women and men and how they can affect access to and control over resources

In the following box, explain and justify which subpopulation(s) the review team has prioritized for further analysis and to be considered in the redesign.

STEP 3

STEP 3 OUTPUTS

Congratulations, the review team has completed the analysis for Step 3!

The review team should **summarize the outputs of Step 3 in a short report (approximately two to five pages)**, while this analysis is fresh in your minds. The output summary should clearly and succinctly capture the main findings and decisions of the review team across the activities in this step. You will be using these output summaries from across the steps towards the end of the review process in Step 7 to bring it all together for the redesign proposal and in a final report on the review process.

The output summary for Step 3 should cover the following components:

• Description of the subpopulations identified in the programme.

• Description of key findings about how these subpopulations have differential health needs and differences in access and benefit of the programme, referring to specific qualitative and quantitative data where possible.

• A revised programme diagram showing which subpopulations are not accessing or benefiting at each key stage of the programme.

• Indication of which subpopulation(s) of the programme were prioritized for further analysis, and an explanation/justification for this.

REFERENCES

Adler NE et al (1994). Socioeconomic status and health: the challenge of the gradient. American Psychologist. 1994;49:15–24.

Alvarez-Dardet C, Montahud C, Ruiz MT (2001). The widening social class gap of preventive health behaviours in Spain. The European Journal of Public Health. 2001;11(2)225–226.

CDC (2013). Potentially Preventable Hospitalizations – United States, 2001–2009. Morbidity and Mortality Weekly Report. Atlanta, Georgia: Centres for Disease Control and Prevention. 2013:62(03);139–143. Available: http://www.cdc.gov/mmwr/preview/mmwrhtml/su6203a23.htm (accessed 22 February 2016).

CSDH (2008). Closing the gap in a generation: Health equity through action on the social determinants of health. Final Report of the Commission on Social Determinants of Health. Geneva: World Health Organization. Available: http://whqlibdoc.who.int/publications/2008/9789241563703_eng.pdf (accessed 22 February 2016).

De Spiegelaere M, Dramaix M, Hennart P (1996). [Social inequalities and prevention: vaccination status of adolescents]. Revue d'epidemiologie et de sante publique. 1996;44(3):228–236.

Eckersley R, Dixon J, Douglas B (2001). The social origins of health and wellbeing. Cambridge University Press.

Galobardes B, Shaw M, Lawlor DA, Lynch JW, Davey Smith G (2006). Indicators of socioeconomic position (part 1). Journal of Epidemiology and Community Health. 2006;60(1):7–12. doi: 10.1136/jech.2004.023531.

Jurges H, Avendano M, Mackenbach JP (2008). Are different measures of self-rated health comparable? An assessment in five European countries. European Journal of Epidemiology. 2008;23(12):773–81. doi: 10.1007/s10654-008-9287-6.

Krieger N (2001). A glossary for social epidemiology. Journal of Epidemiology and Community Health. 2001;55(10):693–700. doi: 10.1136/jech.55.10.693.

Krieger N, Williams DR, Moss NE (1997). Measuring social class in US public health research: concepts, methodologies, and guidelines. Annual Review of Public Health. 1997;18:341–78. doi: 10.1146/annurev.publhealth.18.1.341.

Mackenbach JP, Kunst AE (1997). Measuring the magnitude of socio-economic inequalities in health: an overview of available measures illustrated with two examples from Europe. Social Science & Medicine. 1997;44(6):757–71. Available: http://www.ncbi.nlm.nih.gov/pubmed/9080560 (accessed 22 February 2016).

Ministerio de Salud, Chile (2010). Documento Técnico I, II, III: Serie de Documentos Técnicos del Rediseño de los Programas desde la Perspectiva de Equidad y Determinantes Sociales. Santiago:

Subsecretaría de Salud Pública. [Ministry of Health, Chile (2010). Technical documents I, II and III for supporting the review and redesign of public health programmes from the perspective of equity and social determinants of health. Santiago: Undersecretary for Public Health.] Materials in Spanish only.

Solar O (2014). Presentation overview of the review and redesign process. WHO meeting in Alicante, Spain. June 2014.

Solar O, Irwin A (2010). A conceptual framework for action on the social determinants of health. Social Determinants of Health Discussion Paper 2 (Policy and Practice). Geneva: World Health Organization. Available: http://www.who.int/sdhconference/resources/ConceptualframeworkforactiononSDH_eng.pdf (accessed 22 February 2016).

Tudor Hart J (1971). The Inverse Care Law. Lancet 1971;297(7696):405–12. Available: http://www.sciencedirect.com/science/article/pii/S014067367192410X (accessed 22 February 2016).

United Nations (1948). Universal Declaration of Human Rights, 10 December 1948, 217 A (III).

United Nations (1966). International Convention on the Elimination of All Forms of Racial Discrimination. Treaty Series, 660, 195.

United Nations (1979). Convention on the Elimination of All Forms of Discrimination against Women. New York, 18 December 1979. G.A. res. 34/180, 34 U.N. GAOR Supp. (No. 46) at 193, U.N. Doc. A/34/46, entered into force 3 September 1981.

UN CESCR (Committee on Economic, Social and Cultural Rights) (2009). General Comment No. 20: Non-Discrimination in Economic, Social and Cultural Rights, 02 July 2009, E/C.12/GC/20. Available: http://www.refworld.org/docid/4a60961f2.html (accessed 8 March 2016).

van Doorslaer E, Wagstaff A, van der Burg H et al (2000). Equity in the delivery of health care in Europe and the US. Journal of Health Economics. 2000;19(5):553–583.

van Doorslaer E, Koolman X, Jones AM (2004). Explaining income-related inequalities in doctor utilisation in Europe. Health Economics. 2004;13(7):629–647.

van Doorslaer E, Masseria C, the OECD Health Equity Research Group Members (2004). Income-related Inequality in the Use of Medical Care in 21 OECD Countries. In: Towards High-Performing Health Systems: Policy Studies. Paris: Organisation for Economic Co-operation and Development.

Vega J (2011). Steps towards towards the health equity agenda in Chile. World Conference on Social Determinants of Health, Río de Janeiro, 2011. Available: http://www.who.int/sdhconference/resources/draft_background_paper25_chile.pdf (accessed 22 February 2016).

WHO (2011). Gender mainstreaming for health managers; a practical approach. Geneva: World Health Organization. Available: http://www.who.int/gender-equity-rights/knowledge/health_managers_guide/en/ (accessed 22 February 2016).

WHO (2013). Handbook on health inequality monitoring – with a special focus on low- and middle-income countries. Geneva: World Health Organization. Available: http://apps.who.int/iris/bitstream/10665/85345/1/9789241548632_eng.pdf (accessed 22 February 2016).

WHO (2014). Monitoring health inequality: An essential step for achieving health equity. Geneva: World Health Organization. Available: http://apps.who.int/iris/bitstream/10665/133849/1/WHO_FWC_GER_2014.1_eng.pdf?ua=1 (accessed 22 February 2016).

WHO (2015). State of inequality: Reproductive, maternal, newborn and child health. Geneva: World Health Organization. Available: http://www.who.int/gender-equity-rights/knowledge/state-of-inequality/en/ (accessed 3 March 2016).

STEP 3

Step⁴

Identify the barriers and facilitating factors that subpopulations experience

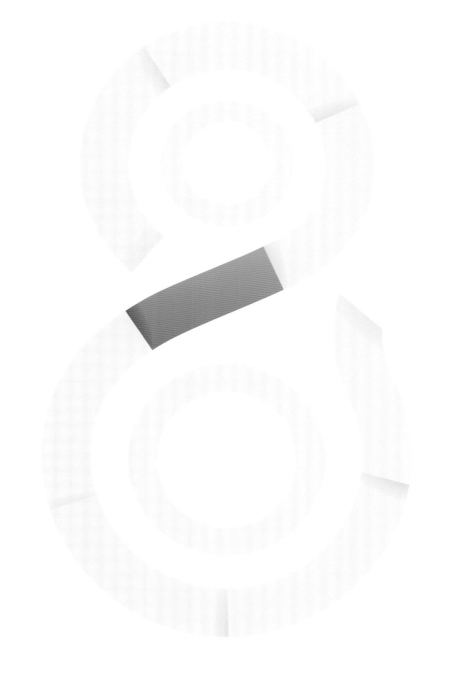

Overview

In Step 4, the review team identifies the barriers and facilitating factors in relation to accessing and benefiting from the health programme. Building on the identification in Step 3 of subpopulations that do not access the programme or may benefit less, the aim in Step 4 is to explore the reasons why these subpopulations do not obtain the anticipated programme results.

To examine the presence or absence of barriers and facilitating factors, Step 4 applies the Tanahashi model of effective coverage – which explores availability, accessibility, acceptability and quality (AAAQ). The four activities of Step 4 guide the review team towards:

1) Assessing the barriers and facilitating factors for the prioritized subpopulation and identification of relevant available data sources;

2) Identifying the most significant barriers at each key stage of the programme and how these limit programme results;

3) Identifying the factors that are facilitating access and benefit at each key stage; and

4) Systematizing the barriers and facilitating factors and developing a revised version of the programme diagram reflecting these findings.

While the previous step tested the programme theory by considering for whom the programme is working and for whom it is not, this step starts to explore *in which contexts and why the programme is not working for them*. It does this by identifying the existence of barriers and facilitating factors and exploring how these function. Step 4 uses information from the work in the previous steps. In particular, it builds on checklist questions on differential needs and living and working conditions, and on considerations related to the enjoyment of the right to health using the AAAQ framework.

The main output of Step 4 is the identification of the main barriers and facilitating factors affecting the subpopulations in the key stages of the programme, which may be integrated in a revised version of the programme diagram (that was developed in Step 2).

Objectives of Step 4

> Understand the Tanahashi model of effective coverage and its links to the AAAQ of the right to health.

> Identify the barriers hindering access and attainment of benefits by priority subpopulation(s) at each key stage of the programme, including gender-related barriers.

> Identify factors that facilitate access and attainment of programme benefits in each key stage for the priority subpopulation(s).

BACKGROUND READING FOR STEP 4

The Tanahashi framework for effective coverage

This reading provides a basic orientation for considering how the priority subpopulation´s problems of not accessing or benefiting less from the programme are related to barriers and facilitating factors. The text covers:

• Tanahashi framework for effective coverage;

• Tanahashi framework's links to the elements of the right to health, i.e. availability, accessibility, acceptability and quality (AAAQ);

• Concepts of barriers and facilitating factors; and

• Summary table with examples of barriers and facilitating factors.

Tanahashi framework for effective coverage

The framework proposed by Tanahashi in 1978 examines programme coverage as a series of dimensions that the beneficiary population must traverse in order to reach effective coverage and obtain the expected benefits. Effective coverage is defined as: "people who need health services obtain them in a timely manner and at a level of quality necessary to obtain the desired effect and potential health gains" (WHO, 2015). Effective coverage is an important concept when considering universal health coverage (UHC) (Evans et al, 2013).

The percentage of the target population with effective coverage depends on the coverage reached in the dimensions of availability, accessibility, acceptability, contact and, finally, effectiveness (see Figure 4.1). The framework aims to identify the target population that is left behind at each step (those left behind are shown by the coverage curve and the box that represents those who do not contact the services).

Figure 4.1 Tanahashi framework for effective coverage

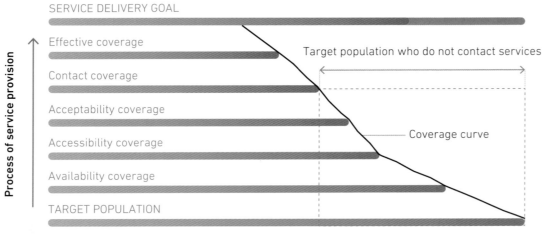

SERVICE DELIVERY GOAL

Process of service provision

Effective coverage

Target population who do not contact services

Contact coverage

Acceptability coverage

Coverage curve

Accessibility coverage

Availability coverage

TARGET POPULATION

Source: Tanahashi, 1978.

Tanahashi framework's links to availability, accessibility, acceptability and quality

The Tanahashi dimensions of availability, accessibility and acceptability provide a useful framework to assess the enjoyment of the right to health (UN CESCR, 2000). Likewise, the notion of service provision of appropriate 'quality' defined in General Comment 14 is also reflected in Tanahashi, with quality-related elements incorporated into the effective coverage dimension and others. Box 4.1 includes extracts from General Comment No. 14 on the Right to the Highest Attainable Standard of Health (UN CESCR, 2000), and provides explanations of the content of these components.

Box 4.1 Availability, accessibility, acceptability and quality as key compoments of a right to health (General Comment No. 14)

General Comment No. 14 on the Right to the Highest Attainable Standard of Health states that all health services, goods and facilities must be available, accessible, acceptable and of good quality (UN CESCR, 2000). The terms availability, accessibility, acceptability and quality are known as **AAAQ** and are featured in the Tanahashi framework, together with stages of contact and, ultimately, effective coverage.

Availability: Functioning public health and health-care facilities, goods and services, as well as programmes, have to be available in sufficient quantity. The precise nature of the facilities, goods and services will vary depending on numerous factors, including the State's level of development. They will include, however, the underlying determinants of health, such as safe drinking-water and adequate sanitation facilities; hospitals, clinics and other health-related buildings; trained medical and professional personnel receiving domestically competitive salaries; and essential drugs. The availability of services can be affected by how decision-makers choose to allocate resources, based on their political priorities or vested interests.

Accessibility: Health facilities, goods and services have to be accessible to everyone without discrimination, within the jurisdiction of the State. Accessibility has four overlapping dimensions: non-discrimination, physical (geographic) accessibility, economic accessibility (affordability) and information accessibility.

Acceptability: Health facilities, goods and services must be respectful of medical ethics and culturally appropriate. This includes being respectful of the culture of individuals, minorities, peoples and communities; sensitive to gender and life-cycle requirements; as well as designing services to respect confidentiality and improve the health status of those concerned.

Quality: Health facilities, goods and services have to be scientifically and medically appropriate and of good quality. This requires skilled medical personnel; scientifically approved and unexpired drugs and hospital equipment; safe and potable water; and adequate sanitation, among other inputs. Issues such as a strong referral network, as well as attention to issues such as treatment adherence, diagnostic accuracy and provider compliance, are important for quality in the context of effective coverage.

Source: UN CESCR, 2000.

It can be noted that the HRBA principle of non-discrimination and equality needs to be considered across AAAQ; this association helps identify barriers that some subpopulations may experience across the dimensions of coverage. There follow some examples of how discrimination based on sex, gender, ethnicity or other characteristics can influence AAAQ.

• **Discrimination and availability:** Some subpopulations may be less represented in decision-making, and hence face indirect discrimination. As a result, consideration of their needs may be less reflected in service prioritization. For example, services for health problems predominantly impacting poor, rural and marginalized subpopulations (e.g. neglected tropical diseases) may be prioritized to a lesser extent than those impacting the middle and upper urban classes in some contexts, as the latter may have more voice in decision-making (WHO, 2012). This will result in availability barriers.

• **Discrimination and accessibility:** Discrimination linked to gender norms, roles and relations can result in men and women having differential access to financial resources, or control over how resources are used, which will affect their experience of the financial accessibility of services.

As mentioned, in the Tanahashi framework, "quality" is not a separate dimension. It is represented by sub-components such as diagnostic accuracy, provider compliance, working referral systems (effective coverage dimension), availability of necessary inputs (availability dimension), perceived responsiveness of provider and perceptions on the quality of care (acceptability dimension). Quality is essentially a cross-cutting feature that underpins the other dimensions in the Tanahashi framework.

Concepts of barriers and facilitating factors

The Tanahashi framework is useful for identifying the reasons why some subpopulations are accessing and benefiting and others are not, at each stage of the programme. It does this by facilitating identification of barriers and facilitating factors.

• **Barriers:** Under this model, barriers are understood as those factors impeding/obstructing the target population (or segment of it) from accessing a programme or making appropriate use of the health service offered. The barriers decrease the effective theoretical coverage of a service, which means that the outcome is only obtained by some specific subpopulations. Accordingly, the programme's impact on the population is less than expected and it generates and perpetuates situations of inequity.

• **Facilitating factors:** These are factors that enable the target population (or segment of it) to make appropriate and full use of the programme, including those that help overcome access barriers and problems of effective use.

It can be noted that often both barriers and facilitators are influenced by the health system and the wider context in which people live, work and age, as well as the interface between these. When they are related to the health system, barriers are sometimes referred to as "supply-side bottlenecks"; when they are linked to wider contextual issues, they can be called "demand-side barriers". Often, impediments to effective coverage represent a combined effect of supply and demand constraints. For instance, a person who lives in a rural area may not receive effective coverage because of the rural remoteness and associated transportation issues, *and* the reality that the service provider network is weak in rural areas and there are no rural mobile/outreach units in place.

With regard to gender, it is important to consider how gender norms, roles and relations can result in both supply-side and demand-side barriers, for instance through lack of availability of same-sex providers or through limited autonomy/decision-making capacity to seek services (WHO, 2011).

Summary table of barriers or facilitating factors in relation to coverage dimensions

Table 4.1 provides an overview of the Tanahashi dimensions and the types or barriers and facilitating factors that can be associated with each. It is not exhaustive, but can be referred to by the review team for guiding analysis.

Table 4.1 Dimensions of Tanahashi framework (including those related to quality) and examples of barriers or facilitating factors

Dimension	Examples of barriers or facilitating factors
Availability	Resources available for delivering an intervention and their sufficiency, namely: • Number or density of health facilities (or outreach services) • Availability of services for different diseases/health topics, as appropriate for population burden of disease (men and women, across the continuum) • Availability of adequately skilled personnel • Availability of necessary inputs (e.g. drugs, equipment)
Accessibility	Geographic: • Distance, availability of transport, time for transportation Financial: • Direct: out-of-pocket expenditures (e.g. co-payment, medicines) • Indirect: opportunity costs (e.g. lost work, child care), transport costs Organizational and informational: • Attention schedules/opening times • Systems to schedule appointments • Administrative requirements for care • Appropriate information sources on health topic, services, treatment Discrimination in access
Acceptability	• Cultural beliefs • Gender-responsiveness of services (including same-sex provider where culturally appropriate) • Age-appropriateness of services (e.g. adolescent-friendly) • Extent to which confidentiality is protected and stigmatization avoided • Perceptions of service quality • Discriminatory attitudes by providers (e.g. based on sex, ethnicity, marital status, religion, caste, sexual orientation)
Contact	• Actual contact between the service provider and the user, similar to "utilization"
Effective coverage	• Barriers in **treatment adherence** (due to unclear instructions, poor patient-provider relationship, mismatch of treatment prescribed with patient compliance ability, adverse social conditions and gender roles/relations preventing follow up by the patient, etc.) • Barriers in **provider compliance** (which can be related to low levels of training, lack of supportive system requirements, absenteeism or other accountability issues, as well as a weak referral and back-referral system) • Barriers in **diagnostic accuracy** (which can be linked to insufficient inputs at health centres and in the laboratory network)

Sources: Tanahashi, 1978; UN CESCR, 2000; WHO, 2010.

STEP 4

Step 4 Additional reading and resources

Tanahashi T (1978). Health service coverage and its evaluation. Bulletin of the World Health Organization. 1978;56(2):295–303. Available: http://www.ncbi.nlm.nih.gov/pubmed/96953 (accessed 22 February 2016).

UN CESCR (Committee on Economic, Social and Cultural Rights) (2000). General Comment No. 14: The Right to the Highest Attainable Standard of Health (Art. 12 of the Covenant), 11 August 2000, E/C.12/2000/4. Available: http://www.refworld.org/docid/4538838d0.html (accessed 4 March 2016).

CASE STUDY EXAMPLE OF STEP 4 FROM A COUNTRY PROGRAMME APPLICATION

This example draws from the colorectal cancer screening programme of the Basque Government of Spain. The programme barriers and facilitating factors for key stages of the screening programme were developed by the review team. Figure 4.2 is an illustrative example of Step 4.

Figure 4.2 Barriers and facilitating factors for key stages of the colorectal cancer screening programme for prioritized subpopulations

Identify and contact participant: Delivery of fecal occult blood test (FOBT) sample in health-care centre	Suspected diagnosis of colorectal cancer: General Practitioner (GP) and nurse consultation with positive FOBT	Confirmation of diagnosis of colorectal cancer

BARRIERS

Availability: The programme is currently only available in 33% of Basque Autonomous Community health-care centres.	**Availability:** The programme is currently only available in 33% of Basque Autonomous Community health-care centres.
Social / cultural accessibility: • Difficulties understanding and interpreting the invitation letter for disadvantaged groups not mastering Basque / Spanish. • Less priority given to possible (forthcoming) health-related problems compared to other actual (current) and greater problems. **Physical accessibility / opening hours:** • Large distance between the health-care centre and the place of residence and work. • Difficulty reconciling working hours with two consultations (GP and nurse).	**Physical accessibility / opening hours:** • Large distance between the health-care centre and the place of residence and work. • Large distance between the hospital and certain geographic areas. • Difficulty reconciling working hours with two consultations (GP and nurse). • For diagnosis confirmation, great difficulty reconciling working hours due to the need to ask for permits.

Acceptability:
• Lesser risk perception and less comprehensive health-care among men.
• Lack of knowledge and awareness of the disease.
• The programme intervenes in aspects that can be seen to interfere with values associated with male identity and the concept of mens' bodies and their management.
• Fear of positive result and lack of knowledge of how to manage it.
	Acceptability:
	• Fear of diagnostic testing and positive confirmatory test.
	• Although it will have less impact than the previous phase, it is worth considering:
	  - Lesser risk perception and less comprehensive health-care among men.
	  - Rejection of colonoscopy due to the type of intervention involved.

FACILITATING FACTORS

Accessibility: • No need for appointment. • Flexible hours in most of the health-care centres (continuous morning and afternoon timetables). • No need to make the delivery in person. • Reminders addressed to people not delivering samples. • Toll-free telephone line providing a continuous information service about the programme.	**Accessibility:** • Possibility of choosing the timetable for the GP and nurse consultation.
Acceptability: • Delivery of the letters according to a geographical schedule that may encourage neighbours talking with each other about the programme, which may increase its acceptability. • Toll-free telephone line providing a continuous information service about the programme.	**Acceptability:** • Toll-free telephone line providing a continuous information service about the programme. • The programme revolves around the health-care centre so that either GPs or nurses can solve doubts and provide health-care advice.

Source: Ministry of Health, Social Services and Equality, Spain, 2012; Portillo et al, 2015; Esnaola, 2015

STEP 4

IDENTIFY THE BARRIERS AND FACILITATING FACTORS THAT SUBPOPULATIONS EXPERIENCE
STEP 4

STEP 4 ACTIVITIES SUMMARY

Table 4.2 contains the activities for the review team to finalize Step 4. It also indicates the questions that orient the activities and the methods used.

Table 4.2 Summary of activities to develop Step 4: Identify the barriers and facilitating factors that subpopulations experience

Questions	Activity components	Methods
Activity 1: Review the Tanahashi framework and identify data sources on barriers and facilitating factors for the prioritized subpopulations		
What is the experience of the identified subpopulation in relation to the dimensions of Tanahashi and which data sources provide information on related barriers and facilitators?	• Review of Tanahashi framework in relation to the prioritized subpopulation(s) and key stages. • Identify potential data sources relevant to the barriers and facilitators faced by priority subpopulations across programme stages.	Review team reflection Analysis of additional data sources Review team discussion
Activity 2: Identify barriers faced by the prioritized subpopulation(s)		
What are the most significant barriers experienced by the priority subpopulation at each stage? How do they limit the programme results?	• Identify specific barriers faced by the priority subpopulation(s) at each key stage of the programme, including gender norms, roles and relations and how they affect access to and control over resources. • Explain how these barriers limit programme access and outcomes.	Review team reflection Data analysis and interpretation Review team deliberation
Activity 3: Identify factors that facilitate accessing and benefiting from the programme		
What are the factors that facilitate accessing and benefiting from the programme at each key stage?	• Identify specific facilitating factors of the programme at each key stage, both for the priority subpopulation(s) and subpopulations who are accessing/benefiting to a greater extent.	Review team reflection Data analysis and interpretation Review team deliberation

Questions	Activity components	Methods
Activity 4: Systematize the barriers and facilitating factors		
What is the summary of main barriers and facilitating factors and how can these be reflected in the programme diagram?	• Summarize the barriers and explain how they limit the interventions in each key stage of the programme, including gender norms, roles and relations and how they affect access to and control over resources. • Summarize the facilitating factors and explain how they strengthen the interventions in each key stage of the programme. • Produce a revised version of the programme diagram with barriers and facilitating factors integrated, including gender norms, roles and relations and how they affect access to and control over resources. • Drawing from the analysis of barriers, reflect if any changes need to be made to the prioritization of the subpopulations and key stages.	Review of concepts and literature Review team deliberation

STEP 4

STEP 4 ACTIVITY GUIDE

The aim of Step 4 activities is to identify the barriers and facilitating factors in relation to accessing and benefiting from the health programme. Using the Tanahashi framework, the review team should – for every stage of the programme – consider barriers and facilitating factors for the following coverage dimensions (in which quality is embedded) (see the background reading section):

- Availability;
- Accessibility;
- Acceptability;

- Contact; and
- Effective coverage.

The review team is reminded that quality considerations span multiple coverage dimensions, and that issues related to direct and indirect discrimination (based on gender, sex, ethnicity, socioeconomic status, etc.) will also influence multiple coverage dimensions. Demand and supply-side factors need to be considered. Please review the background reading for additional details.

ACTIVITY 1

Review the Tanahashi framework and identify data sources on barriers and facilitating factors for the prioritized subpopulations

To carry out this step, it is important to start by considering what are the sources of information available to the review team regarding barriers experienced by the priority subpopulations. The sources can address barriers related to the programme and/or difficulties of access for similar programmes. Sources to be considered include available quantitative data, particularly for the availability, accessibility and contact dimensions. For acceptability, the information is usually qualitative, and is based on the reflexive discussion of the review team. For effective coverage (inclusive of its quality dimensions), the data sources are usually mixed. The experience of the review team members will be central to this analysis, together with consultation with additional programme operators or providers, representatives from the subpopulations (e.g., through focus groups) and the collection of studies that analyse information on interventions with similar theories.

1. **Please list the main sources that the review team will use in its analysis of barriers and facilitating factors for the prioritized subpopulations.**

ACTIVITY 2

Identify barriers faced by the prioritized subpopulation(s)

2. For the key stages of the programme and priority subpopulations (identified in previous steps), the review team should identify the barriers, including in relation to gender norms, roles and relations for women and men and how they affect access to and control over resources. The review team should be as precise as possible in this mapping of barriers. If the review team has identified more than one subpopulation for analysis, *the exercise needs to be done for each subpopulation.* The reason for this is that it will enable the review team to identify the barriers across the stages that are inhibiting programme effectiveness (e.g. attainment of programme outputs and outcomes) as well as impacting health equity and attainment of the right to health.

Barriers to accessing and obtaining benefits – prioritized subpopulation

Subpopulation			
Stage of programme	Barrier	How does the barrier limit the programme results?	Source (review team reflection, programme data, studies, etc.)

ACTIVITY 3

Identify factors that facilitate accessing and benefiting from the programme

The same exercise as that above should be reproduced, focusing on the facilitating factors. That said, this time the exercise should be done for both the prioritized subpopulation and the segments of the overarching target population that have greater access and better outcomes as a result of the programme.

3.a. For the key stages of the programme and priority subpopulations, identify the facilitating factors for the prioritized subpopulations.

Facilitators for access and obtaining benefits – prioritized subpopulation

Subpopulation			
Stage of programme	Facilitator	How does it contribute to improved programme performance?	Source (review team reflection, programme data, studies, etc.)

3.b. For the key stages of the programme and priority subpopulations, identify the facilitating factors for the prioritized subpopulations.

Facilitators for access and obtaining benefits – for subpopulations with better coverage and outcomes

Subpopulations with better access/outcomes			
Stage of programme	Facilitator	How does it contribute to improved programme performance?	Source (review team reflection, programme data, studies, etc.)

ACTIVITY 4

Systematize the barriers and facilitating factors

4. In this final activity, the review team should:

- Discuss the relationship of the identified barriers and facilitating factors with the programme stages that the review team identified in Step 2.

- Revise the programme stages diagram of the key stages generated by the review team in Step 2 (*Understand the programme theory*), incorporating the

main barriers and facilitating factors at key stages. Figure 4.3 provides an example of this.

- Considering the barriers that were identified and the key stages, either confirm or change the prioritization regarding the subpopulation(s) prioritized for analysis.

Figure 4.3 Example: Barriers to cervical cancer screening programme for the prioritized subpopulation

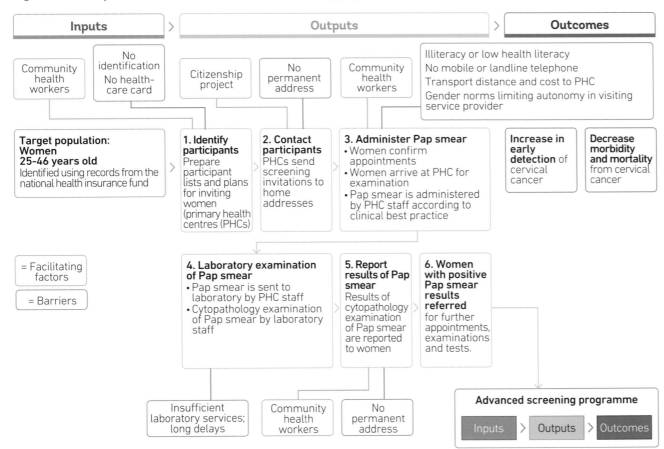

Source: Developed by the authors drawing from WHO Regional Office for Europe, 2015.

IDENTIFY THE BARRIERS AND FACILITATING FACTORS THAT SUBPOPULATIONS EXPERIENCE
STEP 4

STEP 4 OUTPUTS

Congratulations, the review team has completed the analysis for Step 4!

The review team should **summarize the outputs of Step 4 in a short report (approximately two to five pages)**, while this analysis is fresh in your minds. The output summary should clearly and succinctly capture the main findings and decisions of the review team across the activities in this step. You will be using these output summaries from across the steps towards the end of the review process in Step 7 to "bring it all together" when considering your redesign proposals and in a final review team report on the review process.

The output summary for Step 4 should cover the following components:

• Description of the key barriers faced by the prioritized subpopulation(s) and how these limit programme results, referring to specific qualitative and quantitative data where possible. The description should consider gender norms, roles and relations for women and men and how they affect access to and control over resources.

• Description of the key facilitating factors for access and benefits of the programme and how these contribute to improved programme performance, referring to specific qualitative and quantitative data where possible.

• A revised programme stages diagram showing the main barriers and facilitators at each key stage.

• Any adjustments to the prioritized subpopulations of the programme, that the team will apply in the next steps.

REFERENCES

Evans D, Hsu J, Boerma T (2013). Universal health coverage and universal access. Editorial in the Bulletin of the World Health Organization. 2013;91:546–546A. Available: http://www.who.int/bulletin/volumes/91/8/13-125450/en/index.html (accessed 22 February 2016).

Ministry of Health, Social Services and Equality, Government of Spain (2012). Methodological guide to integrate equity into health strategies, programmes and activities. Version 1. Madrid. Available: http://www.msssi.gob.es/profesionales/saludPublica/prevPromocion/promocion/desigualdadSalud/jornadaPresent_Guia2012/docs/Methodological_Guide_Equity_SPAs.pdf (accessed 17 February 2016).

Portillo I, Idigoras I, Bilbao I, Hurtado JL, Urrejola M, Calvo B, Mentxaka A, Hurtado JK (2015). Programa de cribado de cáncer colorectal de euskadi. Centro Coordinador del Programa de Cribado, Subdirección de Asistencia Sanitaria, Dirección General de Osakidetza, Bilbao. Available: http://www.osakidetza.euskadi.eus/contenidos/informacion/deteccion_cancer/es_cancer/adjuntos/programa.pdf (accessed 17 February 2016).

Esnaola S (2015). Les résultats du processus de revue en 5 étapes : cas de la détection précoce du cancer colorectal au Pays Basque (Espagne). Équipe de travail: Bacigalupe A, Aldasoro E, Nuin B, Zuazagoitia J, Millán E, Portillo I, Esnaola S. Presentation at meeting Intégration de l'équité en santé, les déterminants sociaux de la santé, le genre et le droit à la santé atelier de formation sur l'approche «cinq etapes», Rabat, Morocco, 5 November 2015.

Tanahashi T (1978). Health service coverage and its evaluation. Bulletin of the World Health Organization. 1978;56(2):295–303. Available: http://www.ncbi.nlm.nih.gov/pubmed/96953 (accessed 22 February 2016).

UN CESCR (Committee on Economic, Social and Cultural Rights) (2000). General Comment No. 14: The Right to the Highest Attainable Standard of Health (Art. 12 of the Covenant), 11 August 2000, E/C.12/2000/4. Available: http://www.refworld.org/docid/4538838d0.html (accessed 4 March 2016).

WHO (2010). Equity, social determinants and public health programmes. Geneva: World Health Organization. Available:

http://whqlibdoc.who.int/publications/2010/9789241563970_eng.pdf (accessed 22 February 2016).

WHO (2011). Human rights and gender equality in health sector strategies: How to assess policy coherence. Geneva: World Health Organization. Available: http://www.ohchr.org/Documents/Publications/HRandGenderEqualityinHealthSectorStrategies.pdf (accessed 22 February 2016).

WHO (2012). Why are some tropical diseases called "neglected"? Q&A. See: http://www.who.int/features/qa/58/en/ (accessed 22 February 2016).

WHO (2015). Tracking universal health coverage: First global monitoring report. Geneva: World Health Organization. Available: http://apps.who.int/iris/bitstream/10665/174536/1/9789241564977_eng.pdf?ua=1 (accessed 22 February 2016).

WHO Regional Office for Europe (2015). Review and reorientation of the Serbian national programme for early detection of cervical cancer towards greater health equity. Roma health – case studies series no. 3. Copenhagen. Available: http://www.euro.who.int/__data/assets/pdf_file/0011/283646/WHO-Roma-Health-Case-Study_low_V7.pdf?ua=1 (accessed 22 February 2016).

STEP 4

Step 5

Identify mechanisms generating health inequities

Overview

In Step 5, the review team uncovers and understands the relationships and mechanisms operating behind the barriers and facilitating factors in the context in which the priority subpopulations live and where the programme carries on. Completing Step 5 will help the review team articulate why inequities occur in programme access and benefits.

The five activities of Step 5 aim at:

1) Linking barriers and facilitating factors to intermediary and structural social determinants of health;

2) Identifying pathways and mechanisms generating inequities through structural and intermediary determinants;

3) Describing social stratification mechanisms affecting the prioritized subpopulation(s);

4) Identifying how legislation and macro and micro policies influence the social stratification mechanisms or the consequences of socioeconomic position in relation to health inequities and the programme; and

5) Producing a statement of the theory of inequities (i.e. reasons there are inequities) related to the programme access and results.

In completing the activities, the review team will draw on the outputs of the previous steps, as well as any available programme documents, evaluations, studies and other relevant information.

The main output of this step is the statement of *the theory of inequities for the programme*, which explains why inequities occur in relation to programme access and benefits. This helps identify the potential key entry points and opportunities for adjusting the programme to better address these coverage and equity gaps and is the basis for developing the redesign proposal.

Objectives of Step 5

> Apply the WHO conceptual framework of the social determinants of health to understand the mechanisms through which the barriers and facilitating factors act as or are influenced by social determinants.

> Understand how the socioeconomic position of the prioritized subpopulation(s) inter-relates with the barriers and facilitating factors, as well as structural and intermediary social determinants of health.

> Understand the pathways through which the mechanisms generating inequities operate, with regard to differences in exposure, vulnerability and consequences experienced by the prioritized subpopulation(s).

> Understand how discrimination based on sex, gender and other grounds influence social position, driven by social norms and values at the level of structural determinants.

> Identify the theory of inequities of the programme and be aware of the conceptual difference with the theory of the programme from Step 2.

> Consider potential and initial entry points for strengthening an equity, gender, human rights and social determinants focus in the programme, for further exploring in the subsequent steps.

IDENTIFY MECHANISMS GENERATING HEALTH INEQUITIES STEP 5

BACKGROUND READING FOR STEP 5

Understanding the mechanisms generating health inequities

This background reading focuses on the mechanisms and pathways associated with the generation of health inequities. It sheds light on the "causes of the causes" behind inequities in relation to the programme. In Step 5, "why" is explored in relation to:

• The "base" for inequities that a person has according to their social position, linked to their levels of prestige, resources and experience with discrimination (due to gender, ethnicity, caste, etc);

• Pathways through which inequities manifest themselves linked to differential exposure, differential vulnerability and differential consequences;

• Intermediary and structural determinants of health (as illuminated in the WHO conceptual framework of the social determinants of health (Solar & Irwin, 2010) to portray causality and thus produce a synthesis of "theories of health inequities"; and

• Theories on the social causation of health inequities that underpin the pathways and mechanisms.

These issues are explained both in the reading and in the supplementary reading built into the activities for Step 5.

While there are some common drivers of inequities for all programmes and countries, it is necessary to consider the specificities of a particular programme and the local and national context. In some countries, public policies, programmes and interventions can mitigate inequities through the existence of programmes that support the most vulnerable or more disadvantaged subpopulations. Other actions may address the more structural causes of inequities, as well as intervene at the whole society level, making it more feasible to eliminate inequities. Yet, on the other hand, some policies and programmes may deepen or widen inequities, making it even harder to overcome them. For this reason, it is important for health programme managers to understand the "whys" behind inequities, so that a theory of inequities can be identified and the programme can take that into account in its efforts to reduce them.

Introduction to causal mechanisms behind health inequities

Differences in health based on income, place of residence (rural/urban), sex, education or occupation are well established, varying between countries. Various models based on theories of causation, selection and their modifications have been proposed to explain these differences, but the reasons and mechanisms involved are still not properly understood (Bartley, 2004).

One of the first attempts to unravel causal mechanisms was the Black Report (Black et al, 1980). The approach adopted in the report represented the traditional explanation where what the report termed as

"socioeconomic health inequalities"[1] derive from two main mechanisms: the **selection mechanism** and the **causation mechanism**. However, it was soon argued that although important, causation and selection as such would not suffice to explain socioeconomic differences in health (Bartley et al, 1998).

A social causation perspective suggests that socioeconomic position has an effect on health through unequal distribution of determinants of health across social groups. **Socioeconomic position** is defined

---

[1] This Innov8 Technical Handbook uses the WHO approach of differentiating "health inequities" (avoidable or unfair differences in health status or in the distribution of health determinants between different population groups) and "health inequalities" (measures of these differences, using stratifiers, e.g. income, education, which may or may not be avoidable or unfair). However, the term "health inequalities" is sometimes used interchangeably with the term "health inequities", as is the case in the Black Report referenced here.

and modelled in large part by the **sociopolitical and economic context**, which acts to buffer or aggravate social conditions generated by social stratification and/or social exclusion. Socioeconomic position influences health through more specific determinants of health and illness, which can be called **intermediary determinants**. Various intermediary social determinants of health will have a different role in specific programmes: in some the role of psychosocial aspects is fundamental, yet for others material and housing conditions or the labour market are centre stage. These differences must be explored in the review process, since they are crucial to understanding the main causes of inequities and to identifying effective interventions to integrate in order to strengthen equity, gender, human rights and social determinants issues in the programme.

Multiple and complex causal mechanisms are often used to explain socioeconomic differences in health. Indeed, in the debate and discussion that followed the publication of the Black Report researchers began to consider the possibility of more complex mechanisms, including the effect of psychosocial factors as well as the development of health inequities over the life course and the influence of political economy (Bartley et al, 1998).

Socieconomic position: base of the mechanism

Socioeconomic position refers to the social and economic factors that influence the position that *individuals or groups* have within the structure of a society. Socioeconomic position is understood to be an aggregate concept that includes integrated measurement of access to resources and prestige in society, linking to social class (Marx, Weber, Krieger, Williams and Moss) (Solar & Irwin, 2010).

Socioeconomic position has effects of poorer material conditions on health (for example poor housing or work-related conditions and hazards) or relative deprivation (where people assess their own socioeconomic position in relation to others, irrespective of absolute affluence).

Finally, socioeconomic position has a strong relation with the distribution of power in society (Solar & Irwin, 2010), and the distribution of power is associated with resources, prestige, as well as discrimination:

- **Resource-based** mechanisms of stratification refer to access to material and social resources, including income and salary. The term "health inequities" is used when resources are insufficient and inadequate and there are situations of poverty and deprivation.

- **Prestige-based** mechanisms of stratification refers to individual ranking or status in the social hierarchy, and is typically evaluated in terms of the magnitude and quality of access to and consumption of goods, services and knowledge. Today, in many cultures, prestige is associated with occupation, income and educational level.

- **Discriminatory-based** mechanisms of stratification – for example, as mentioned in earlier chapters, "gender" refers to those characteristics of women and men/girls and boys which are socially constructed, whereas "sex" designates those characteristics that are biologically determined. Gender involves "culture-bound conventions, roles and behaviours" that shape relations between and among women and men and boys and girls (Borrell et al, 2014:31; WHO, 2011a). In many societies, gender norms, roles and relations contributes to unequal power relations that shape the ability of men and women to make choices and take actions to be healthy.

STEP 5

Box 5.1 The "base" of the mechanism

When unpacking the causes of the causes of health inequities in a given subpopulation, start by considering socioeconomic position or social stratification. Do so by considering factors including:

- Level and unequal distribution of social prestige;
- Level and unequal distribution of resources; and
- The discrimination that they may experience (based on gender, ethnicity, caste or other factors).

IDENTIFY MECHANISMS GENERATING
HEALTH INEQUITIES STEP 5

It is likely that the origin of health inequities lies partly in the fact that people in lower socioeconomic groups live and work in circumstances that may have a detrimental effect on health. The behavioural explanation indicates that those in lower socioeconomic positions have poorer health due to health-damaging behaviours (smoking, drinking, physical inactivity, infrequent use of health care, etc.), which can be more common in lower socioeconomic groups in some countries. Researchers emphasize that differences in morbidity and mortality cannot be entirely explained by well-known behavioural or material risk factors of disease. An example is in "cardiovascular disease outcomes, where risk factors such as smoking, high serum cholesterol and blood pressure can explain less than half of the socioeconomic gradient in mortality" (Mackenbach & Bakker, 2002:13).

Behavioural factors, such as smoking, diet, alcohol consumption and physical exercise, are certainly important determinants of health. Patterns differ significantly from one country to another. For example, in 1998 smoking was generally more prevalent among lower socioeconomic groups; however, in southern Europe, smoking rates were higher among higher income groups, and in particular among women (Cavelaars et al, 1998). The contribution of diet, alcohol consumption and physical activity to health inequities is less clear and not always consistent. However, there is a higher prevalence of obesity and excessive alcohol consumption in lower socioeconomic groups, particularly in richer countries.

Role of the health system in relation to health inequities

The health system itself constitutes an additional relevant intermediary factor, though one which has often not received adequate attention in the literature on social determinants. The role of the health system in influencing health inequities is particularly important when considering availability, accessibility, acceptability and effective coverage (the domains covered in the previous step), acknowledging that these are the combined result of both supply-side issues and demand-side factors. Differences in access to quality health services, across the continuum, certainly do not fully account for the social patterning of health outcomes. Adler and Newman (2002) considered the role of access to health services in explaining the health gradient according to socioeconomic position and concluded that access alone could not explain the gradient. The health system can directly try to reduce exposure to risk factors and vulnerability to ill health, as well as improve equitable and non-discriminatory access to health services. It can promote intersectoral action to act on wider social and environmental determinants of health and improve health status. Examples of the latter would include food supplementation, in conjunction with the food and agricultural sector, and transport policies that can help overcome

geographic barriers to access health and other critical social services.

A further aspect of great importance is the role the health system plays in mediating the differential consequences of illness in people's lives. As supported by WHO work on universal health coverage, financial risk protection can facilitate that health problems do not lead to impoverishment or catastrophic health expenditures. The health system can also help prevent stigmatization as a result of ill health and facilitate people's social reintegration after illness. Examples of social reintegration include programmes for the chronically ill to support their reintegration in the workforce. Benzeval et al (1995) argue that the health system has three obligations in confronting inequity:

- To ensure that resources are distributed between areas in proportion to their relative needs;

- To respond appropriately to the health-care needs of different subpopulations; and

- To take the lead in encouraging a wider and more strategic approach to developing healthy public policies at both the national and local level, to promote equity in health and social justice.

Main emerging theories on the causes of health inequities in social epidemiology

The main theoretical directions currently invoked by social epidemiologists for understanding the causes of health inequities are: materialist or neo-materialist; cultural psychosocial approaches; life course; political economy; and ecosocial theory. These are not mutually exclusive.

All these approaches explain the "causes of the causes" and mechanisms driving health inequities, which they presume cannot be reduced to conventional theories of disease causation. Where they differ is in their respective emphasis on different aspects of social and biological conditions in shaping population health, how they integrate social and biological explanations, and thus their recommendations for action.

Table 5.1 summarizes the main explanations for the relationship between wider social inequalities (e.g. income inequality) and health inequities described in the literature. As noted, these explanations are not exclusive, and the relative importance of one or another explanation is given by the context and the type of problem addressed. It is important when reading each of the explanations to analyse their relevance in relation to the programme being reviewed.

Table 5.1 Main theories explaining the relationship between social inequalities and health inequities

	Explanation types	Examples
Materialist/ neo-materialist	The effect of income inequality on health reflects both lack of resources held by individuals and systematic under-investments across a wide range of community infrastructure. The links between income inequality and health must begin with the structural causes of inequalities, and not just focus on perceptions of that inequality. Thus, income inequality per se is but one manifestation of a cluster of material conditions that affect population health.	Individual income determines access to a healthy diet, quality housing, an unpolluted environment, better working conditions, good education, etc.
Cultural/ behavioural	From this point of view, socioeconomic gradients in health are the result of social class differences in behaviours such as poor diets, consumption of tobacco or alcohol, the absence of exercise or underuse of preventive health care (vaccination, prenatal controls, screening). This approach is favoured by doctors and health professionals and, often is mistakenly taken to imply that such behaviours are largely under individual control. Nevertheless, even though the evidence supports the causal significance of these behaviours, they are conditioned by the social and material context in which they occur. Thus, rather than being independent causes, behaviours are intervening variables between social structure and illness (Blane et al, 1997).	Differences in beliefs, norms and values – including gender norms, roles and relations – mean that women and men, boys and girls from less advantaged social groups in some countries are less likely to drink alcohol moderately, more likely to use tobacco and less likely to exercise in leisure time. While cultural and religious values ("traditions") often provide material and psychosocial support to people through access to social capital and networks, some gender norms, roles and relations maintain pressure on women and girls to drop out of school, marry young, initiate childbearing soon after marriage, or have numerous and closely spaced pregnancies to add status to the family or ensure a male heir.

	Explanation types	Examples
Psychosocial	According to this view, people's perception and experience of personal status in unequal societies leads to stress and poor health. The experience of living in social settings of inequality forces people constantly to compare their status, possessions and other life circumstances with those of others. This engenders feelings of shame and worthlessness in people experiencing disadvantage, along with chronic stress that undermines health. The two different pathways from stress to health are first, the direct effect of stress on disease development and, second, an indirect route where stress leads to health damaging behaviours. At the level of society as a whole, meanwhile, steep hierarchies in income and social status weaken social cohesion; with this disintegration of social bonds also seen as negative for health.	Status, control, social support at work or at home, and the balance between effort and reward influence health through their impact on body functions. The psychosocial perspective supports the idea that psychosocial pathways are associated with relative disadvantage, which adds to the direct effects of absolute material living conditions.
Life course	A life-course approach explicitly recognizes the importance of time and timing in understanding causal links between exposures and outcomes within an individual life course, across generations, and in population-level diseases trends. Two main mechanisms are identified. The "critical periods" model is when an exposure acting during a specific period has lasting or lifelong effects on the structure or function of organs. This is also known as biological programming and is also sometimes referred to as a latency model. This conception is the basis of hypotheses on the fetal origins of adult diseases and does recognize the importance of later life effect modifiers, for example in the linkage of coronary heart disease, high blood pressure and insulin resistance with low birth weight. The "accumulation of risk" model suggests that factors that raise disease risk or promote good health may accumulate gradually over the life course, although there may be developmental periods when their effects have greater impact on later health than factors operating at other times. This idea is complementary to the notion that as the intensity, number and/or duration of exposures increase, there is increasing cumulative damage to biological systems.	Events and processes starting before birth and during childhood may influence both physical health and the ability to maintain health. Health and social circumstances influence each other over time. Risk factors tend to cluster in socially patterned ways. For example, those living in adverse childhood social circumstances are more likely to be of low birth weight, and be exposed to poor diet, childhood infections and passive smoking. These exposures may raise the risk of adult respiratory disease, perhaps through chains of risk or pathways over time where one adverse (or protective) experience will tend to lead to another adverse (protective) experience in a cumulative way.

	Explanation types	Examples
Political economy	Economic processes and political decisions condition the private resources available to individuals and shape the nature of public infrastructure – education, health services, transportation, environmental controls, availability of food, quality of housing, occupational health regulations – that forms the "neo-material" matrix of contemporary life.	Political processes and distribution of power affect the provision of services, quality of the physical environment and social relationships. Countries and regions in which economic and social resources are better distributed have better health indicators. This suggests that better redistribution of resources is critical. Examples of this include labour market resources such as employment; welfare state resources such as health-care coverage and public health expenditures, education, family supportive services, and social transfer resources; cultural resources such as civil associations; and political resources such as the distribution of power.
Ecosocial	The ecosocial approach and other emerging multi-level frameworks have sought to integrate social and biological reasoning and a dynamic, historical and ecological perspective. In this context, Krieger's (2001a) notion of "embodiment" is an especially important concept "referring to how we literally incorporate biologically influences from the material and social world in which we live, from conception to death; a corollary is that no aspect of our biology can be understood absent knowledge of history and individual and societal ways of living".	More than simply adding "biology" to "social analysis", or "social factors" to "biological analyses", the ecosocial framework begins to envision a more systematic integrated approach capable of generating new hypotheses.

Elaborated by the authors from: Solar & Irwin, 2010; WHO, 2010.

STEP 5

IDENTIFY MECHANISMS GENERATING HEALTH INEQUITIES STEP 5

The pathways of the mechanisms that produce health inequities

According to Diderichsen (1998) and as further elaborated by other authors and WHO (Solar & Irwin, 2010; WHO, 2010), the mechanisms through which socioeconomic position relays differentials in health outcomes operate through three pathways.

> ### Box 5.2 Pathways through which the mechanisms for inequities operate
>
> - Differential exposure;
> - Differential vulnerability; and
> - Differential consequences.

- **Differential exposure:** Exposure to most risk factors (material, psychosocial and behavioural) is inversely related to social position. Many health programmes do not differentiate exposure or risk reduction strategies according to social position. Evidence suggests that people in disadvantaged positions are subject to differential exposure to a number of risk factors, including anthropogenic crises, unhealthy housing, dangerous working conditions, low food availability and quality, social exclusion and barriers to adopting health behaviours.

- **Differential vulnerability:** The same level of exposure may have different effects on different social groups, depending on their social, cultural and economic environments and cumulative life course factors. Clustering of risk factors in some population groups, such as social exclusion, low income, alcohol abuse, malnutrition, cramped housing and poor access to health services may be as important as the individual exposure itself. Co-existence of other health problems, such as co-infection, often augments vulnerability.

- **Differential consequences:** Poor health may have several and different social and economic consequences, including loss of earnings, loss of ability to work and social isolation or exclusion. Further, sick people often face additional financial burdens that render them less able to pay for health care and drugs. Population groups who may experience more advantage are better protected, for example in terms of job security and health insurance. For those who may experience disadvantage, however, ill health might result in further socioeconomic degradation, crossing the poverty line and accelerating a downward spiral that further damages health. Due to gender roles, women and girls in households are often expected to shoulder the burden of home-based care-giving responsibilities for family members, in addition to their other activities.

When considering a theory of inequities, it is important to think of the pathways through which inequities are generated. Social stratification engenders differential exposure to health-damaging conditions and differential vulnerability, in terms of health conditions and material resource availability. Based on their relative social positions, individuals and groups experience: unequal exposures to health risks, differential vulnerability as a result of these unequal exposures; and differential social, economic and health consequences as a result of these unequal exposures and vulnerabilities. These differences increase with time, and are often transmitted from generation to generation (WHO, 2008).

How the mechanisms and pathways generating inequities are portrayed in the WHO conceptual framework of the social determinants of health

The WHO conceptual framework of the social determinants of health is described in detail in the *Introduction to applied concepts, principles and frameworks*. This framework draws from multiple theories of causation mentioned above in the Table 5.1. The framework makes a distinction between structural and intermediary determinants, emphasising the difference between social determinants of health inequities and social determinants that influence health. Implicit in the original framework are also the pathways leading to the differentials in exposure, vulnerability and consequences. The adapted version of the framework (Figure 5.1) highlights more explicitly how these pathways work in relation to intermediary determinants of health. Only by understanding the mechanisms and pathways of these structural and intermediary determinants and their interaction with the programme and the target population is it possible to comprehend why the programme works or fails and for whom.

Figure 5.1 Summary of mechanisms and pathways presented in the conceptual framework of the social determinants of health, WHO

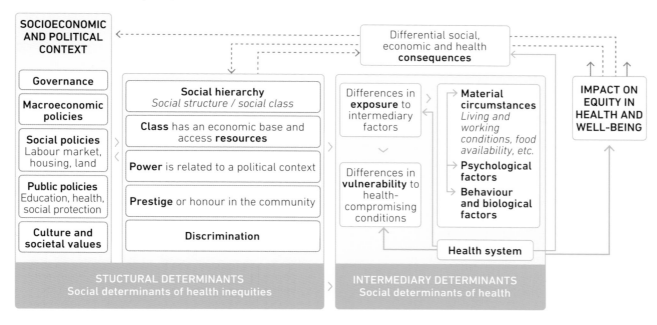

Source: Solar & Irwin, 2010.

Gender in relation to the causal mechanisms behind health inequities

This section will deepen the *cultural explanation*, which has great relevance when analysing social values and norms, and how these translate into discriminatory actions at individual, community and societal levels. It does so by considering how gender-linked health inequities are generated. Gender involves "culture-bound conventions, roles and behaviours" that shape relations between and among women and men and boys and girls (Krieger, 2001b:694; Borrell et al, 2014; WHO, 2011a). In many societies, gender constitutes a fundamental basis for discrimination, which can be defined as the process by which members of a socially defined group are treated differently, especially unfairly because of their inclusion in that group.

Gender is a crucial and strong determinant of most health outcomes (Krieger, 2003; CSDH, 2007; WHO, 2011a). Differentials often exist between men and women across health conditions, related to sex and gender. Unlike men and women's biological characteristics, gender is a social construct, defining cultural conventions, roles, behaviours and relationships between and among women and men, which vary from society to society and across generations and may be changed. From birth, women and men, boys and girls are taught norms and roles thought to be appropriate by the majority in their community, including how men and women are supposed to behave, how they should relate and their roles in families, communities and the workplace. Gender shapes differences between women and men, boys and girls in exposure to disease and injury, household-level investment in nutrition, care and education, access to and use of health services and social impact of ill-health. Gender can enable or constrain the ability of men and women to make choices and lead healthy lives. Gender interacts with other sociocultural characterstsics, including stigma, discrimination and social exclusion faced by individuals or groups of women and men, and may adversely affect health. A gender analysis of health identifies and assesses these mechanisms to provide evidence to inform actions to address gender inequalities in health, including how biological (sex) and sociocultural (gender) factors interact to influence health behaviour, outcomes and services for women and men, boys and girls.

Borrell et al (2014:13) remarked that:

> "The acquisition of gender roles and stereotypes starts early with the socialization of girls and boys, continues throughout the life course, and results in gender inequalities in power and in the unequal division of paid and unpaid work. On the one hand, patriarchy, the systematic domination of women by men, restrains women's access to social and employment-related privileges and economic resources and assigns them a larger share of domestic responsibilities (unpaid work) with consequences to women's health status. Hegemonic masculinity, on the other hand, understood as the development and maintenance of a heterosexual male identity, promotes the taking of risks that are hazardous to health and contributes to premature mortality among men compared with women Thus, although biology plays a part in health differences between men and women, the higher burden of suffering is related mainly to social inequalities grounded in gender."

Several epidemiologic studies show that gender-linked health inequities are shaped by inequalities between men and women in key social determinants of health, including: (i) economic dependence and income differences as a consequence of differential access to labour markets, segregation or gendered pay gaps, and, resulting in elderly women in limited entitlement to pensions; (ii) paid work by women is less valued (horizontal segregation), they wield less authority (vertical segregation), and face other differentials in working conditions; and (iii) unpaid work, when gender ideology attaches to women primary responsibility for domestic labour performed in the household, including care for others (Borrell et al, 2014).

Macrosocial or structural determinants of health, such as political power, welfare state and social protection policies, and economic and labour market policies, are the major drivers of the social structure and power relations within society. These power relations generate health inequities that researchers are investigating, including their causal roots and the policy responses (welfare state, social protection, economic and labour market policies) that increase or reduce social and health inequities (Marmot et al, 2010). In this perspective, it is important to analyse more deeply the wider contexts in which programmes develop. Figure 5.2 presents an overview to help the review team examine the ways that contextual factors influence gender inequities, with the view towards understanding different levels of policy intervention, ranging from individual, family to community and societal.

Figure 5.2 Policies for gender equality

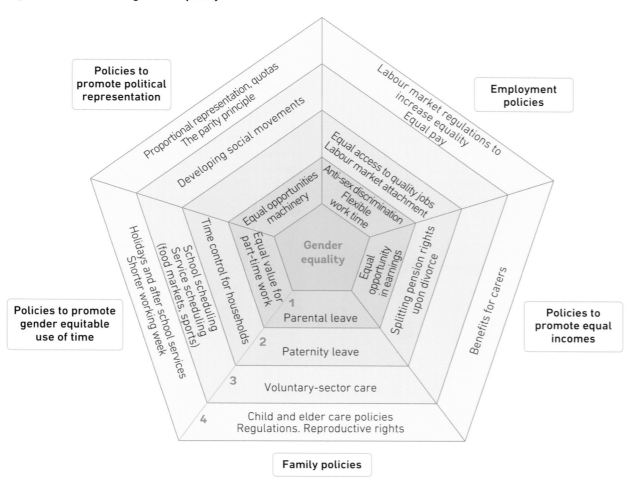

Note: Levels of policy intervention – 1 individual; 2 household; 3 civic/community; 4 society/political.

Source: Reproduced from Carme Borrell et al. Influence of Macrosocial Policies on Women's Health and Gender Inequalities in Health. Epidemiologic Reviews (2014) 36 (1): 31-48 (Fig. 1 & PP. 32-34 [291 words]). By permission of Oxford University Press on behalf of the Johns Hopkins Bloomberg School of Public Health. Modified from Pascall & Lewis, 2004.

While often beyond the direct or indirect control of the health sector, a number of social and economic policies have the potential to contribute to reducing gender-linked health inequities, particularly women´s health, according to Borrell et al (2014). It is important that the review team is cognizant of these entry points to address "causes of the causes" of gender-linked health inequities and gender-linked barriers to services.

• **Policies to promote political representation:** Women, compared with men, often have fewer opportunities to be socially and politically active and to influence laws and politics. Some policies to increase women's participation in politics include proportional representation and quotas to reach greater representational parity. Policies aimed at developing social movements that advocate for women's interests are also important.

• **Employment policies:** Men often benefit from more opportunities for paid work and better employment conditions. Gender equality policies should also promote equal access to quality jobs. In many cases, gendered employment policies seek to give men and women flexible work time so they can reconcile paid work with family and civil society activities.

• **Policies to promote equal incomes:** Men and women have unequal access to income. This relates mainly

STEP 5

to the fact that women often have less access to paid work, worse paid jobs, lower salaries for the same jobs and, consequently, lower pensions. Other policies that have been instituted in this area include equal rights to benefits (e.g. pensions), taking into account that pensions for women are lower as unpaid care and work are not taken into account nor are pensions appropriately split upon divorce.

- **Family policies:** This group of policies seeks to increase family well-being and to promote reconciliation between paid work and family. Family support is a cross-cutting issue that may include support for employment, transportation, food, education, and so on.

- **Policies to promote gender-equitable use of time:** Women have less time than men because they often bear a greater burden of unpaid work. Policies that promote less gender-biased uses of time are policies that produce time control in the household, to develop the different activities. Anti-gender discrimination policies for the labour market are useful, but part-time work should have equal value to full-time work.

Moreover, the framing of social justice and equity, points towards the adoption of related human rights frameworks as vehicles and fundamental values for enabling the full realization of the right to health, for which the State is the primary responsible duty bearer (WHO, 2011b).

Step 5 Additional reading and resources

CSDH (2007). Unequal, Unfair, Ineffective and Inefficient. Gender Inequity in Health: Why it exists and how we can change it. Final report to the WHO Commission on Social Determinants of Health.

WHO (2011a). Gender mainstreaming for health managers: a practical approach. Geneva: World Health Organization. Available: http://whqlibdoc.who.int/publications/2011/9789241501071_eng.pdf (accessed 24 February 2016).

WHO (2011b). Human rights and gender equality in health sector strategies: How to assess policy coherence. Geneva: World

Health Organization. Available: (http://www.ohchr.org/Documents/Publications/HRandGenderEqualityinHealthSectorStrategies.pdf (accessed 24 February 2016).

WHO (2011c). Closing the gap: Policy into practice on social determinants of health. Discussion paper. Geneva: World Health Organization. Available: https://extranet.who.int/iris/restricted/bitstream/10665/44731/1/9789241502405_eng.pdf (accessed 24 February 2016).

CASE STUDY EXAMPLE OF STEP 5 FROM A COUNTRY PROGRAMME APPLICATION

Outputs from the review of Chile´s cardiovascular health programme have been presented in previous chapters. Here, we present the results of the review team's work in linking the barriers and facilitating factors to the intermediary and structural social determinants and the underlying mechanisms of action that are operating to generate inequities.

The review team´s analysis identified that the programme provided inadequate coverage to men aged between 45 and 64 years, with the main excluded groups being workers with social risk factors such as low education, unstable or precarious employment and low-income residents and workers in poorer districts **(prioritized subpopulations).**

The **socioeconomic position** of this subpopulation was found to be associated with increased exposure, vulnerability and deleterious health consequences with observed higher rates of morbidity and mortality for ischemic heart disease and stroke. The socioeconomic position of this group is associated with income levels, education, occupation and employment status (temporary and precarious employment). The "cause of the causes" is the distribution of resources, prestige and discrimination for this social group. **This is a key structural determinant.**

The other **key structural determinants** found were associated with macroeconomic and social policies, in particular with regard to employment conditions and tax redistribution, as well as low income and low educational level. Some remarks and examples relating to social policies are presented in Table 5.2.

The **key intermediary determinants** analysed by the review team included *psychosocial* beliefs and myths associated with chronic diseases and stress. The *health-care system care* itself was also one of the obstacles to access to health care, primarily due to the rigid/inflexible opening hours of health-care centres and services and the high turnover of staff. The health-care system does not recognize the heterogeneity of the population and needs, nor the context of this group: it does not see workers in the target population. In addition, material conditions such as working conditions and employment are key intermediary determinants that impact directly on the health of this group and limit the access to the health service. Examples are given in Table 5.2.

Theory of inequities: The primary care centre-based programme with a biomedical focus offered during working hours, limited access by working people. The lack of a gender perspective and community and workplace outreach, was particularly limiting for men. The organization of consultations was not coordinated to facilitate adherence, requiring multiple visits both for inscription and regular controls. The limited coverage of social policies increases the vulnerability of this subpopulation. To address inequities in this subpopulation requires intervention in the organization of the health system, but also in labour market conditions.

Table 5.2 Linkages between the barriers and facilitating factors and the intermediary and structural social determinants and the underlying mechanisms generating inequities

Barrier or facilitating factors identified in Step 4	Social determinants link with barriers	Mechanism of actions of social determinants	How mechanism works (review the different theories)
Barrier Organization and management of health-care services	Health-care system	Opening hours hinder access and adherence to the programme for working people (especially rigid schedules). Heterogeneity of population and differential need not recognized. Indifferent, passive and low empathy health teams, who lack the skills to promote and sustain protective behavioural changes for health (discrimination).	*Culture* of the health-care system: Biomedical programme focus, with limited health system permeability *Materialist theory*: Restriction of the human resources and time schedule in the health-care system
Barrier Precarious conditions of employment and work	Psychosocial factors Material circumstances	Experiences and difficult life management and sense of helplessness with regard to possible intervention situations. The priority of this group is the satisfaction of basic needs (food, housing, and clothing). Demanding attention only at point of emergency; seeking preventive actions are not prioritized in daily lives.	*Materialist theory*. *Political economy* in relation to regulation of welfare state to the temporary worker and regulation of the labour market
Barrier Low risk perception, resistance to behaviour changes, low motivation toward prevention	Behavioural factors	Habits and risk behaviour generate greater exposure, vulnerability and negative health consequences. Lack of supportive networks.	*Cultural behavioural theory* *Psychosocial theories*
Barrier Low level of schooling and income	Material circumstances Psychosocial factors	Low income and precarious employment conditions limit access and adherence. Perception of risk and health-seeking behaviour limit contact with the health system.	*Political economy* *Psychosocial theory*
Facilitator Programmes on social protection	Social policies Health system policies	Act by reducing the vulnerability of those with greatest disadvantage. (But, as these are not universal, they leave out some groups experiencing relative disadvantage.)	*Political economy*

Sources: Ministerio de Salud, Chile, 2010; Solar, 2014; Analysis of equity in the access and outcomes of the cardiovascular health programme and its relation with the Social Determinants of Health Work Team: National Node of Cardiovascular Health General Coordination: Dr María Cristina Escobar, Dr Johanna Silva EU Marina Soto.

STEP 5 ACTIVITIES SUMMARY

Table 5.3 contains the activities and the components of each activity that the review team will develop to finalize Step 5. It also indicates the questions that orient the activities and the methods used.

Table 5.3 **Summary of activities to develop Step 5: Identify mechanisms generating health inequities**

Questions	Activity components	Methods
Activity 1: Linking barriers and facilitating factors to intermediary and structural social determinants of health		
How do the barriers act as or are associated with social determinants of health, including gender, in relation to the programme for the priority subpopulation(s)?	• Analyse the social determinants linked to the barriers and facilitating factors in the key stages of the programme identified in the previous step.	Review team reflection Data analysis and interpretation Review team deliberation
Activity 2: Pathways and mechanisms generating inequities through structural and intermediary determinants		
What are the pathways and mechanisms between the structural and intermediary determinants linked to the barriers and facilitating factors?	• Description of the mechanisms related to the structural and intermediary social determinants which explain the presence of barriers and facilitating factors to access that affect the prioritized subpopulation(s) and act on health inequities.	Review team reflection Data analysis and interpretation Review team deliberation
Activity 3: Social stratification mechanisms affecting the prioritized subpopulation(s)		
What are the social stratification mechanisms that determine the socioeconomic position of the prioritized subpopulation(s), considering resources, prestige and discrimination?	• In-depth characterization of prioritized subpopulation(s) in relation to socioeconomic position linked to social stratification mechanisms, integrating quantitative and qualitative data.	Review team reflection Analysis of additional data sources Review team discussion
Activity 4: Identify how macro and micro policies and legislation influence social stratification mechanisms or the consequences of socioeconomic position in relation to health inequities and the programme		
How do relevant public policies and legislation affect or influence the priority subpopulation(s) in relation to health inequities and programme access and benefits?	• Analysis of macroeconomic policies/strategies, social policies and legislation that affect the subpopulation and influence health programme results. • Identify and analyse other health sector programmes that impact positively or negatively on the programme in review.	Review team knowledge and reflection Analysis of available documents Analysis of additional data sources Review team discussion

STEP 5

IDENTIFY MECHANISMS GENERATING HEALTH INEQUITIES STEP 5

Questions	Activity components	Methods
Activity 5: Write a statement of the theory of inequities (i.e. reasons there are inequities) related to the programme access and results		
Why do inequities in relation to programme access and results occur in the priority subpopulation(s)?	• Write an initial statement of the theory of inequities related to the programme. Review and refine the statement as a starting point for programme redesign.	Review team reflection, drawing on previous steps Review of concepts and literature Review team deliberation and summary

ACTIVITY 1

Linking barriers and facilitating factors to intermediary and structural social determinants of health

To facilitate the work, have Figure 5.3 on hand. This summarizes the conceptual framework used to analyse the social determinants of health and the generation of inequities in health, and highlights the three domains.

Figure 5.3 Conceptual framework of the social determinants of health, WHO

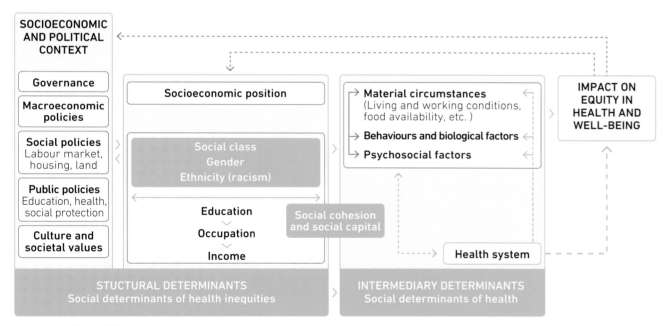

Source: Solar & Irwin, 2010

As noted in the reading, a society is usually stratified according to income, education, occupation, gender, ethnicity and social class, the weighting of each based on the realities of each society, and changing across time and place. A person's socioeconomic position, in turn, defines and influences a number of factors that determine more directly the health status to these factors, and we call them **intermediary determinants of health**. The main categories of intermediary determinants of health are:

- **Material circumstances** that include determinants linked to physical environments, such as housing (including condition, location and the type of neighbourhood); consumption potential, such as funding to purchase healthy food, clothes, working conditions, and the physical environment of the neighbourhood. Depending on the quality of these aspects, these circumstances become resources for access to health or otherwise become health risks.

- **Psychosocial circumstances,** which include psychosocial stressors such as negative life events, stressful living conditions (e.g. high debt or financial insecurity) and lack of social support. Different social groups are exposed throughout their lives to different situations that are perceived as threatening, difficult to manage and/or offering little possibility for intervention. Fear of violence (including gender-based violence), and restricted decision-making autonomy shaped by gender norms, roles and relations, are psychosocial factors that can have an impact on health (CSDH, 2007). This mainly explains the patterns that are associated with long-term health inequities.

- **Behaviour patterns,** which include smoking, diet, alcohol consumption and lack of exercise. Depending on the pattern of exposure and vulnerability they may become protective factors or enhance health, like exercise, or otherwise be harmful to health as with cigarette smoking and obesity. One issue to note is that habits and "lifestyles" are the result of the material conditions in which one is born, lives and works. They are the way that social groups translate the material conditions of life into patterns of behaviour.

- **The health system itself** can directly intervene on the differences in exposure and vulnerability, through equitable access to health care and the promotion of intersectoral action to improve health status. Also, the health system acts as a mediator or buffer to the consequences of an illness or disability on the lives of people by ensuring that the health problem does not result in a deterioration in social status and also facilitate the social reintegration of people with disabilities or illness.

- **Social cohesion,** which considers the set of integration mechanisms that exist in a society, and other perceptions of citizens on the operation of these mechanisms. The latter in turn determine the sense of belonging to a social group by the groups that comprise it. We can say that discrimination is a determinant of social cohesion that justifies government intervention to address it. There is no single definition of **social capital**. However, beyond the range of definitions, there is some consensus that it is an intangible and dynamic resource that exists in the collective and it includes elements such as trust, participation and reciprocity.

In the previous step the review team identified the barriers and facilitating factors, and now analyses their association with intermediary and structural determinants: these are the material conditions, psychosocial factors, behaviours and habits, the system health itself and the social capital (social cohesion) and sociopolitical context.

1.a. The review team should discuss these aspects mapping them in the following tables. Identify each barrier and mark with an 'X' the intermediary social determinants that are associated with it. More than one linked social determinant can be marked for each barrier. The review team should be able to provide an explanation for the association.

Health programme		Intermediary determinants associated with the barrier					
Describe barriers	Associated programme key stage(s)	Material circum-stances (living and working conditions)	Behaviours and habits	Psychosocial factors	Health system factors	Social cohesion/ social capital	Explanation

1.b. Some of the barriers identified might be associated with structural determinants. The review team should examine this in the following table.

Barriers description	Associated programme key stage(s)	Examine the association of the barrier with STRUCTURAL SOCIAL DETERMINANTS (i.e. the health insurance system, gender norms, social protection system)

1.c. The same process should be carried out for the facilitating factors.

Health programme		Intermediary determinants associated with facilitating factor					
Describe facilitating factors	Associated programme key stage(s)	Material circum-stances (living and working conditions)	Behaviours and habits	Psychosocial factors	Health system factors	Social cohesion/ social capital	Explanation

1.d. Some of the facilitating factors identified might be associated with structural determinants. The team should examine this in the following table.

Facilitating factors description	Associated programme key stage(s)	Examine the association of the facilitating factors with the STRUCTURAL SOCIAL DETERMINANTS

ACTIVITY 2

Pathways and mechanisms generating inequities through structural and intermediary determinants

Once the barriers and facilitating factors have been associated with social determinants of health (intermediary and structural), the team will begin the core analysis of Step 5: *What are the possible mechanisms of action to address inequities in programme access and results?*

2. To answer this question, the review team should start by briefly reviewing the concepts introduced in the reading. Then, the review team should consider each of the following questions and document them in the following table.

1. What are the pathways through which the mechanisms generating inequities are occurring:
   a. Differential exposure;
   b. Differential vulnerability;
   c. Differential consequences.

2. Considerering the socioeconomic position of the population as a starting point, what is the "base" of the drivers behind inequities, for instance:
   a. Lesser access to or control over resources;
   b. Lesser levels of prestige;
   c. Discrimination based on sex, gender, ethnicity, or other factors;
   d. A combination of the above (describe).

3. Which of the main theories on the causes of health inequities can best explain the mechanisms driving inequities in relation to the programme:
   a. Materialist or neo-materialist;
   b. Cultural;
   c. Psychosocial approaches;
   d. Life course;
   e. Political economy;
   f. Ecosocial theory

Key stage	Main social determinants of health associated to that barrier of the key stage (draw from previous tables)	Pathway of mechanisms (exposure, vulnerability, consequences)	Base of the mechanism (resources, prestige, discrimination)	How does the mechanism operate (review the theories in the reading and Table 5.1)

Identify the social stratification mechanisms affecting the prioritized subpopulation(s) in relation to their socioeconomic position, including gender issues

3. Based on their combined knowledge and experiences, in this exercise the review team members are asked to discuss and describe aspects of the socioeconomic position of the prioritized subpopulation(s) (identified in Step 3) and the underlying social stratification mechanisms. The questions the team should answer are:

• What is the **socioeconomic position** of the prioritized subpopulation(s) from the perspective of resources, prestige and discrimination, including differences between men/boys and women/girls within that subpopulation, if applicable?

• What are the **social stratification mechanisms** operating that place the subpopulation(s) in this socioeconomic position?

In Step 3 the review team described the socioeconomic position of the subpopulations. In Step 5, the review teams will use of available data will deepen the analysis in relation to social stratification mechanisms such as distribution of power (resources, prestige, discrimination) that have expression in the level of education or income, type of occupation, gender, geographic location, ethnicity, etc.

Reference can be made to how these aspects impact the subpopulations from early in life and accumulate throughout the life cycle and may be reproduced across generations.

The review team's answers to these questions should be briefly summarized in the following box.

Description of the prioritized subpopulation in terms of their socioeconomic position
(i.e. from the perspective of resources, prestige, discrimination, including consideration of differences between men and women/girls and boys *within* that subpopulation if applicable, and highlighting the social stratification mechanisms in place)

IDENTIFY MECHANISMS GENERATING HEALTH INEQUITIES STEP 5

ACTIVITY 4

Identify how legislation and macro and micro policies influence social stratification mechanisms or the consequences of socioeconomic position in relation to health inequities and the programme

Following the analysis of socioeconomic position, the context can be discussed (remember that the socioeconomic position and context are defined in the conceptual framework as the **structural determinants).**

The socioeconomic position is defined and modelled in large part by the sociopolitical and economic context, as they act to buffer social conditions generated by social stratification and/or social exclusion. The context includes the political and policy context:

- **Macroeconomic policies**, including fiscal and monetary balance, fiscal debt and balance of payment, treaties and policies on the labour market.

- **Social policies and related legislation** affecting factors such as labour, property and the distribution of land and housing.

- **Public policies and related legislation** in areas such as education, social welfare, health, water and sanitation.

4.a. Now the review team should analyse legislation, policies or strategies related to the context described in the conceptual framework that would be impacting on the prioritized subpopulation(s) in relation to health inequities and the results of the health programme under review. For each policy selected (at least one) the team should complete the following table.

Name of legislation, public policy or strategy	
How does this legislation or public policy affect or influence the socioeconomic position of the priority subpopulation?	
How does the legislation or policy affect the context in which the health programme is developed?	

Now, the review team should go back to the diagram of the programme theory drawn in Step 2 and consider it in relation to Figure 5.4, which represents the **micro context** where the health programme is being developed. In the below Figure, imagine the team is reviewing programme 2, which is a TB programme. We can see that other programmes and interventions, such as HIV and food security programmes are fundamental to the TB programmes results. On the other hand, competing priorities such as maternal-child programmes may have a negative impact unless synergies between them and the TB programme are developed. Likewise, maternal and reproductive programmes may ignore the specific needs and circumstances of adolescents. To reach this subpopulation, schools and other community interventions are key. Figure 5.4 also emphasises the timeline of influences within the context.

Figure 5.4 Better comprehension of the ecology of interventions

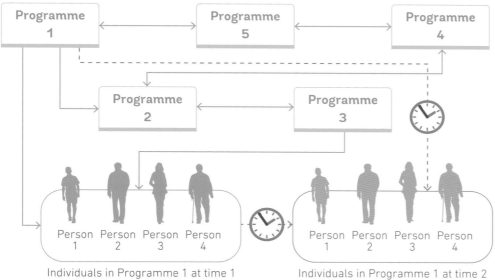

Individuals in Programme 1 at time 1   Individuals in Programme 1 at time 2

Source: Sridharan, 2009.

4.b. Returning to the reality of the programme´s micro context, the team should discuss: What other programmes and interventions are influencing, either positively or negatively, the health programme being reviewed?

Describe each programme and how it interacts with the health programme being reviewed.

Programmes and interventions that influence the health programme being reviewed		
Name of programme or intervention	Description	Interaction with the health programme in review

IDENTIFY MECHANISMS GENERATING HEALTH INEQUITIES STEP 5

ACTIVITY 5

Write a statement of the theory of inequities (i.e. the reasons there are inequities) related to the programme

In Step 2 the review team laid out the programme theory. Now, with the elements from Steps 3 and 4 and Step 5 activities, the review team has identified the mechanisms generating inequities that explain why some subpopulations do not access or benefit and the barriers related to the key stages affecting these subpopulations, which act through social determinants pathways. In this activity, the review team will take these explanations of why inequities occur in relation to accessing and benefiting in different key stages to articulate the theory of inequities of the programme.

5.a. To do this the review team should discuss the following questions:

- Returning to the statement of the programme theory and the programme diagram with the key stages developed in Step 2. **Why does it not work for all subpopulations?**

- In Step 3, by identifying the subpopulations with problems in accessing or benefiting, inequities in relation to the programme were confirmed. **What key stages of the programme are most critical for these populations and why?**

- Then the review team identified barriers (and facilitators) for the subpopulations in the key stages (Step 4) and linked these to social determinants of health (in this Step 5). **Why do these social determinants generate inequities in this subpopulation?**

Considering these questions and the conclusions from the previous exercises, the review team should now try to explain, in three paragraphs, why inequities related to the programme are occurring. This explanation is a statement of the theory of inequities.

Write a statement of the theory of inequities related to the programme.

5.b. Review this statement of the theory of inequities, considering the following questions.

- Does it explain why the initial programme **theory** is insufficient to address equity, gender, human rights and social determinants?

- What assumptions about the programme functioning were wrong and obscured the **mechanisms** generating inequities? For example, if it was assumed all the population had the same need, would all demand services and would all receive them?

- Does it include how the policy **context (macro and micro) generates inequities**?

- Does it consider how **differentials in subpopulation needs** and living conditions determine that the programme works differently?

- Does it consider how **gender norms, roles and relations** influence programme results?

- Does it take into account that the measures to ensure **human rights principles** may be insufficient?

In the light of this discussion revise the statement of the theory of inequities, if necessary, and rewrite.

With this theory of inequities, the review team sets out on the path towards the redesign of the programme and the elaboration of recommendations to strengthen equity, gender, human rights and social determinants perspectives.

STEP 5 OUTPUTS

Congratulations, the review team has completed the analysis for Step 5!

The review team should **summarize the outputs of Step 5 in a short report (approximately two to five pages)**, while this analysis is fresh in your minds. The output summary should clearly and succinctly capture the main findings and decisions of the review team across the activities in this step. You will be using these output summaries from across the steps towards the end of the review process in Step 7 to "bring it all together" in a final review team report on the review process.

The output summary for Step 5 should cover the following components:

• Description of the intermediary and structural determinants associated with the barriers and facilitating factors for the programme that affect the prioritized subpopulation(s).

• Description of the pathways and mechanisms related to these structural and intermediary social determinants, which explain health inequities and the presence of these barriers and facilitating factors.

• Description of the prioritized subpopulation(s) in relation to socioeconomic position (including gender), referencing specific quantitative and qualitative data where possible.

• Description of how relevant public policies affect or influence the priority subpopulation(s) in relation to health inequities and programme access and benefits, including legislation and macroeconomic policies/strategies and social policies as well as the positive or negative influence of other health sector programmes.

• Statement of the theory of inequities related to the programme.

REFERENCES

Adler NE, Newman K (2002). Socioeconomic Disparities in Health: Pathways and Policies. Health Affairs. 2002;21(2):60–76. Available: http://doi.org/10.1377/hlthaff.21.2.60 (accessed 24 February 2016).

Bartley M (2004). Health inequality an introduction to theories, concepts and methods. Cambridge, UK: Polity Press.

Bartley M, Blane D, Davey Smith G (1998). Introduction: Beyond the Black Report. Sociology of Health and Illness. 1998;20(5):563–677.

Benzeval M, Judge K, Whitehead M (1995). Tackling inequalities in health: An agenda for action. London: King's Fund.

Black D, Morris J, Smith C, Townsend P (1980). Inequalities in health: Report of a Research Working Group. London: Department of Health and Social Security.

Blane D, Bartley M, Davey Smith G (1997). Disease aetiology and materialist explanations of socioeconomic mortality differentials. European Journal of Public Health. 1997;7(4):385–391. Available: doi: http://dx.doi.org/10.1093/eurpub/7.4.385 (accessed 7 March 2016).

Borrell C, Palència L, Muntaner C, Urquía M, Malmusi D, O'Campo P (2014). Influence of macrosocial policies on women's health and gender inequalities in health. Epidemiologic Reviews. 2014;36(1):31–48. Available: http://epirev.oxfordjournals.org/content/36/1/31.abstract (accessed 24 February 2016).

Cavelaars AE, Kunst AE, Geurts JJ, Crialesi R, Grötvedt L, Helmert U, Lahelma E, Lundberg O, Matheson J, Mielck A, Mizrahi A (1998). Differences in self reported morbidity by educational level: a comparison of 11 western European countries. Journal of Epidemiology and Community Health. 1998;52(4):219–227.

CSDH (2007). Unequal, Unfair, Ineffective and Inefficient. Gender Inequity in Health: Why it exists and how we can change it. Final report to the WHO Commission on Social Determinants of Health.

Diderichsen F (1998). Understanding health equity in populations — Some theoretical and methodological considerations. In: Arve-Parès B, ed. Promoting research on inequality in health. Stockholm: Socialvetenskapliga Forskningsrådet [Swedish Council for Social Research]:99–114.

Krieger N (2001a). Theories for social epidemiology in the 21st century: an ecosocial perspective. International Journal of Epidemiology. 2001;30(4):668–677.

Krieger N (2001b). A glossary for social epidemiology. Journal of Epidemiology and Community Health. 2001;55(10):693–700.

Krieger N (2003). Genders, sexes, and health: what are the connections – and why does it matter? International Journal of Epidemiology. 2003;32(4):652–657.

Mackenbach J, Bakker M (2002). Reducing Inequalities in Health: A European Perspective. London: Routledge.

Marmot M, Allen J, Goldblatt P, et al (2010). Fair Society, Healthy Lives: Strategic Review of Health Inequalities in England post-2010. London: United Kingdom. The Marmot Review.

Ministerio de Salud (2010). Documento Técnico I, II, III: Serie de Documentos Técnicos del Rediseño de los Programas desde la Perspectiva de Equidad y Determinantes Sociales. Subsecretaría de Salud Pública: Santiago. [Ministry of Health, Chile (2010). Technical documents I, II and III for supporting the review and redesign of public health programmes from the perspective of equity and social determinants of health. Santiago: Undersecretary for Public Health.] Materials in Spanish only.

Pascall G, Lewis J (2004). Emerging Gender Regimes and Policies for Gender Equality in a Wider Europe. Journal of Social Policy. 2004;33(03):373. Available: http://journals.cambridge.org/abstract_S004727940400772X (accessed 24 February 2016).

Solar O (2014). Presentation overview of the review and redesign process. WHO meeting in Alicante, Spain. June 2014.

Solar O, Irwin A (2010). A conceptual framework for action on the social determinants of health. Social Determinants of Health Discussion Paper 2 (Policy and Practice). Geneva: World Health Organization. Available: http://www.who.int/sdhconference/resources/ConceptualframeworkforactiononSDH_eng.pdf (accessed 24 February 2016).

Sridharan S (2009). Ten steps to making evaluation matter. Presentation at Evaluation Workshop, Santiago, Ministry of Health, Chile. Sanjeev Sridharan, University of Toronto and Centre for Urban Health Research at St Michael's Hospital.

Verbrugge LM (1985). Gender and health: an update on hypotheses and evidence. Journal of Health and Social Behavior. 1985;26(3):156–182.

WHO (2008). Closing the gap in a generation: health equity through action on the social determinants of health. Final Report of the Commission on Social Determinants of Health. Geneva: World Health Organization. Available: http://apps.who.int/iris/bitstream/10665/43943/1/9789241563703_eng.pdf (accessed 24 February 2016).

WHO (2010). Equity, social determinants and public health programmes. Geneva: World Health Organization.

WHO (2011a). Gender mainstreaming for health managers: a practical approach. Geneva: World Health Organization. Available: http://whqlibdoc.who.int/publications/2011/9789241501071_eng.pdf (accessed 24 February 2016).

WHO (2011b). Human rights and gender equality in health sector strategies: How to assess policy coherence. Geneva: World Health Organization. Available: (http://www.ohchr.org/Documents/Publications/HRandGenderEqualityinHealthSectorStrategies.pdf (accessed 24 February 2016).

WHO (2011c). Closing the gap: Policy into practice on social determinants of health. Discussion paper. Geneva: World Health Organization. Available: https://extranet.who.int/iris/restricted/bitstream/10665/44731/1/9789241502405_eng.pdf (accessed 24 February 2016).

Step6

Consider intersectoral action
and social participation
as central elements

Overview

In Step 6, the review team considers the role of intersectoral action and social participation as central elements to tackle health inequities in relation to the health programme. The analysis in Step 6 applies concepts and methods held in common from the equity, gender, human rights and social determinants fields. For example, participation is a core principle of a human rights-based approach , and intersectoral action is implicit in the nature of the right to health as an inclusive right that includes a wide range of underlying determinants that influence health.

Regarding intersectoral action, the analysis focuses on how working with other sectors is relevant to addressing the identified coverage gaps, barriers and facilitating factors and related social determinants in the key stages of the programme. For social participation, the goal is to ensure an adequate response to health needs and to empower social groups – particularly the priority subpopulation(s) identified – to achieve better programme access and benefits for all.

Step 6 entails four activities to be conducted in relation to the key stages of the programme under review:

1) Identifying and characterizing intersectoral action to address issues identified in previous steps;

2) Prioritizing and developing or improving intersectoral action;

3) Describing the current approach to social participation by the programme, and

4) Prioritizing and developing/improving actions for social participation that contribute to addressing the barriers and facilitating factors.

These activities integrate findings from the previous steps of the review process, together with available information.

There are two main outputs for Step 6. The first is an assessment of how intersectoral action and social participation are currently functioning in the programme. The second is a proposal or set of recommendations for developing or enhancing intersectoral action and strengthening social participation mechanisms, which will contribute to tackling coverage gaps, barriers and facilitating factors, in order to improve programme access and benefits for all, particularly the priority subpopulation(s).

Objectives of Step 6

> Analyse and apply the concepts and approaches of intersectoral action and social participation to understand how these are currently represented in the programme and how they impact on the programme and its results.

> Identify the role of intersectoral action and social participation in tackling the identified programme barriers and contributing to reducing health inequities, for each stage and for the prioritized subpopulation.

> Identify specific recommendations (inclusive of mechanisms and actions) for strengthening intersectoral action and social participation during the redesign of the health programme, as that will be advanced in the subsequent steps.

BACKGROUND READING FOR STEP 6

The role of intersectoral action and social participation in health programmes

This background reading aims to provide the review team with basic orientations for thinking about the role of intersectoral action and social participation in relation to health programmes to address health inequities, before beginning work on Step 6.

The text covers:

• Intersectoral action and social participation in the framework of tackling social determinants of health inequities;

• Intersectoral action in the development and implementation of a programme; and

• Social participation in the development and implementation of a programme.

Intersectoral action and social participation in the framework of tackling social determinants of health inequities

Many of the most important and powerful influences that shape health and the distribution of health inequities are located outside the health sector (WHO, 2008). That these influences lie outside of the exclusive jurisdiction of the health sector means that the health sector needs to engage and act in collaboration with other sectors of government and society in order to address the determinants of health and well-being (WHO, 2008).

Intersectoral action and **social participation** are two strategic approaches for tackling the social determinants of health inequities, as demonstrated in Figure 6.1, which illustrates different levels or entry points for interventions or actions to address inequities. It also points to the necessity of taking into consideration intersectoral action, and social participation and empowerment, as two central aspects that cross transversally the pro-equity action or programme (Solar & Irwin, 2010).

Figure 6.1 **Framework for tackling social determinants of health inequities**

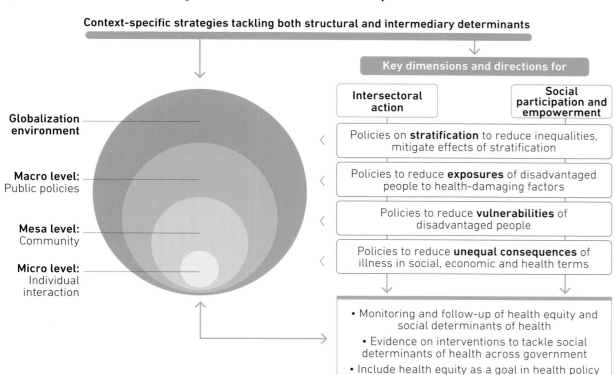

Context-specific strategies tackling both structural and intermediary determinants

Key dimensions and directions for

Intersectoral action	Social participation and empowerment

Policies on **stratification** to reduce inequalities, mitigate effects of stratification

Policies to reduce **exposures** of disadvantaged people to health-damaging factors

Policies to reduce **vulnerabilities** of disadvantaged people

Policies to reduce **unequal consequences** of illness in social, economic and health terms

- Monitoring and follow-up of health equity and social determinants of health
- Evidence on interventions to tackle social determinants of health across government
- Include health equity as a goal in health policy and other social policies

Globalization environment

Macro level: Public policies

Mesa level: Community

Micro level: Individual interaction

Source: Solar & Irwin, 2010.

Intersectoral action refers to actions affecting health outcomes undertaken by sectors outside the health sector, possibly, but not necessarily, in collaboration with the health sector. Intersectoral action for health entails health and other sectors working together to inform public policy design and implementation to improve health and well-being, or, minimally, not to adversely affect it. Such efforts improve understanding across health and other sectors about the way that the policy decisions and operational practices of different sectors impact on health and health equity.

Social participation of civil society and the empowerment of women and men from affected communities to have a greater role in shaping social policy to advance health and health equity are critical from both an ethical and a pragmatic standpoint and a rights perspective. As the underlying basis of inequities is the unequal distribution of power, money and resources, empowerment and meaningful participation constitute one of the mechanisms for the redistribution of power. In this way it can contribute to modifying inequities and give greater space to action and intervention in the existing social hierarchy, both at global level as well as at programme level.

In the same way that inequities are the result of a complex accumulation of disadvantages, interventions often require a network of actions by multiple sectors and at multiple levels. The sequence and coordination of the involvement of other sectors and the level and type of social participation should be part of the analysis of the redesign of the programme.

STEP 6

CONSIDER INTERSECTORAL ACTION AND SOCIAL PARTICIPATION AS CENTRAL ELEMENTS
STEP 6

Intersectoral action in the development and implementation of a programme

Historically, from the public health perspective, a systemic approach to addressing the problems of population health has frequently been advocated, with particular emphasis on the different social, administrative and economic sectors, as well as on the diversity of cultures and values that comprise and stratify societies. Accordingly, health issues – in a broader definition – have boundaries beyond the health sector and the majority of health determinants are largely outside the direct scope of the health sector. These issues are therefore unlikely to be solved by exclusive actions of the health sector.

Air pollution offers one example. One in eight deaths globally is linked to air pollution exposure – mostly from heart and lung disease, and stroke (WHO, 2014a). To tackle air pollution, a health ministry cannot act alone. Collaboration is needed within many sectors, including those responsible for household energy, energy supply, transport, urban planning, housing, waste management, industry, and local, regional and country municipalities. As stated at the 8th Global Conference on Health Promotion, "The health of the people is not only a health sector responsibility; it is a wider political issue" (WHO, 2013).

The concept of intersectoral action is an evolving one, with several waves of development historically. Briefly, these include:

• A call for intersectoral action for health that emerged out of the WHO's Declaration of Alma-Ata (WHO Regional Office for Europe, 1978). This called on the health sector to direct efforts beyond the delivery of acute hospital-based medicine/services towards primary health care and factors underpinning health, in particular, determinants such as water, food, education and housing.

• In the decade following, the 1986 WHO Ottawa Charter for Health Promotion (WHO, 1986) called for healthy public policy, which considers intersectoral action with regard to key health concerns such as environmental challenges, tobacco and alcohol legislation as well as gender inequalities.

• The third wave of intersectoral action for health developed during the Finnish Presidency of the European Union in 2006, wherein the Presidency called upon governments across Europe to ensure that health considerations were to be included in all government policies, coining the phrase "Health in All Policies" (HiAP) (Kickbusch & Buckett, 2010).

A common definition for Health in All Policies (HiAP) is:

> "An approach to public policies across sectors that systematically takes into account the health implications of decisions, seeks synergies, and avoids harmful impacts, in order to improve population health and health equity."
>
> WHO, 2013; World Health Assembly, 2014.

Box 6.1 provides further information about the Health in All Policies approach to intersectoral action.

Box 6.1 Definitions and concepts: Health in All Policies

A strategy that allows the formulation of public policies in sectors other than health, which when applied can correct, improve or positively influence the determinants of health.

A systematic approach to taking into account the impacts of public policies on health determinants, including health systems, in order to realize health-related rights, to seek synergy across sectors and to improve the accountability for the impacts of policies, and ultimately population health and health equity.

An initiative that focuses on influencing the health of the population and its determinants. A central element is cooperation between different relevant sectors within and beyond the domain of public health regarding aspects of health. The common goal is to improve, promote or protect health.

Examples of concepts highlighted as important in the definition:

- Systemic and sustained approaches/strategies
- Intersectoral win-win and efficiency
- Impacting on determinants and health systems
- Reach in public policy or beyond
- Human rights
- Political context and participation
- Importance of communities
- Importance of leadership
- Monitoring the evolution and impact of policies

Source: Compiled from responses to a public web-based consultation, facilitated by WHO, for a working definition for the 8th Global Conference on Health Promotion, 2013; WHO, 2014b.

Intersectoral action refers broadly to the relationships arising between policy sectors across government that require finding appropriate common values, mechanisms and structures to accommodate differences in disciplinary origins, existing organizational culture, political hierarchy and rhetoric in order to deliver better services to the population. These efforts are directed towards actions in both health and other sectors. This **intersectorality** constitutes an essential requirement to address inequities and social determinants of health.

There are several types or levels of intersectoral relationships (Solar et al, 2009; Solar & Cunill, 2015):

- **Relationships based on "information":** The focus is on information exchange between sectors, such as sharing the results of a study or analysis in the sector. This can be considered as a first step in a process of intersectoral work, with information sharing or communication being part of the process of building a common language for achieving dialogue and understanding.

- **Relationships based on "cooperation":** This refers to interaction between sectors to achieve greater

efficiency in the actions of each sector. This usually entails transforming incidental, casual or reactive cooperation into actions strategically oriented to those problems where the activities of other sectors may be decisive. This often means that it is the health sector which leads the initiative. This type of intersectoral action is usually present at the stage of programme or policy enforcement or implementation, rather than during formulation.

- **Relationships based on "coordination":** This entails a joint effort working towards the adjustment of the policies and programmes of each sector for the purpose of greater efficiency and effectiveness. It points to more horizontal networking among sectors and often comprises a shared financing source. These are important components, as creating synergies (or at least to avoiding non-synergies) within public administration requires taking a broader view of the issues or problems at hand. Coordination translates into greater interdependence among the sectors involved and hence also a loss of autonomy for each sector.

- **Relationships based on "integration":** Integrated work involves defining a new policy or programme together with other sectors in a way in which the responsibility and work falls to more than one sector. Integrated intersectoral action also entails the sharing of resources, responsibilities and actions, which therefore necessarily calls for solidarity or power sharing. From this perspective the integration of policies can be simultaneously accompanied by

autonomy of the sectors, since formulation, design and financing of actions are agreed upon and elaborated based on a common social goal rather than on particular sectoral requirements.

Table 6.1 shows the inter-relationships between health and well-being and illuminates the roles of different sectors in this.

Table 6.1 Inter-relationships between health and well-being that illustrate why "joined-up" government action is necessary

Sectors and issues	Inter-relationships between health and well-being
Economy and employment	• Economic resilience and growth is stimulated by a healthy population. Healthier people can increase their household savings, are more productive at work, can adapt more easily to work chances and can remain working for longer. • Work and stable employment opportunities improve health for all people across different social groups.
Security and justice	• Rates of violence, ill health and injury increase in populations whose access to food, water, housing, work opportunities and a fair justice system is poorer. As a result, justice systems within societies have to deal with the consequences of poor access to these basic needs. • The prevalence of mental illness (and associated drug and alcohol problems) is associated with violence, crime and imprisonment.
Education and early life	• Poor health of children or family members impedes educational attainment, reducing educational potential and abilities to solve life challenges and pursue opportunities in life. • Educational attainment for both women and men directly contributes to better health and the ability to participate fully in a productive society, and creates engaged citizens.
Agriculture and food	• Food security and safety are enhanced by consideration of health in food production, manufacturing, marketing and distribution through promoting consumer confidence and ensuring more sustainable agricultural practices. • Healthy food is critical to people's health, and good food and security practices help to reduce animal-to-human disease transmission, and are supportive of farming practices with positive impacts on the health of farm workers and rural communities.
Infrastructure, planning and transport	• Optimal planning for roads, transport and housing requires the consideration of health impacts as this can reduce environmentally costly emissions and improve the capacity of transport networks and their efficiency with moving people, goods and services. • Better transport opportunities, including cycling and walking opportunities, build safer and more liveable communities and reduce environmental degradation, enhancing health.

Sectors and issues	Inter-relationships between health and well-being
Environments and sustainability	• Optimizing the use of natural resources and promoting sustainability can be best achieved through policies that influence population consumption patterns, which can also enhance human health. • Globally, a quarter of all preventable illnesses are the result of the environmental conditions in which people live.
Housing and community services	• Housing design and infrastructure planning that take account of health and well-being (e.g. insulation, ventilation, public spaces, refuse removal, etc.) and involve the community can improve social cohesion and support for development projects. • Well-designed, accessible housing and adequate community services address some of the most fundamental determinants of health for disadvantaged individuals and communities.
Land and culture	• Improved access to land can support improvements in health and well-being for indigenous peoples as indigenous people's health and well-being are spiritually and culturally bound to a profound sense of belonging to land and country. • Improvements in indigenous health can strengthen communities and cultural identity, improve citizen participation and support the maintenance of biodiversity.

Source: Adelaide Statement on Health in All Policies (WHO, Government of South Australia, Adelaide 2010).

The health sector's engagement in intersectoral action for health is in keeping with a human rights-based approach to health. The right to health is an inclusive right (WHO & OHCHR, 2001). It includes a wide range of factors that influence health by acting on underlying determinants. The Committee on Economic, Social and Cultural Rights, the body responsible for monitoring the International Covenant on Economic, Social and Cultural Rights, makes reference to accounting for determinants such as the following in efforts to ensure the right to health (WHO & OHCHR, 2001):

• Safe drinking-water and adequate sanitation;
• Safe food;
• Adequate nutrition and housing;
• Healthy working and environmental conditions;
• Health-related education and information; and
• Gender equality.

As appropriate for the programme under review, the areas/actions identified in this section can be considered in programme planning exercises and relevant intersectoral interventions planned.

Social participation in the development and implementation of a programme

"It is... essential to see the public not merely as 'the patient' whose well-being commands attention, but also as 'the agent' whose actions can transform society".

Drèze & Sen, 1989:279.

Participation is reflected as a **requirement for the attainment of the highest possible level of health of all people** (Potts, 2010). This is reflected in the WHO Constitution (International Health Conference, 1946), Declaration of Alma-Ata (WHO Regional Office for Europe, 1978), Ottawa Charter for Health Promotion

CONSIDER INTERSECTORAL ACTION AND SOCIAL PARTICIPATION AS CENTRAL ELEMENTS
STEP 6

(WHO, 1986) and Rio Political Declaration on Social Determinants of Health (World Conference on Social Determinants of Health, 2011), among others. The importance of a participatory approach is also highlighted in the UN Common Understanding on rights-based approaches and WHO's global strategy and framework on people-centered and integrated health services.

The WHO Commission on Social Determinants of Health identified participatory approaches as a critical component of a health system that had capacity to tackle health inequities (CSDH, 2008). The commission called for *organizational arrangements and practices* that involve population groups and civil society organizations (particularly those working with socially disadvantaged and marginalized groups), in decisions and actions that identify, address and allocate resources to health needs.

Participation is a **cross-cutting principle embodied in international human rights treaties** and the general comments and recommendations adopted by the bodies monitoring their implementation (OHCHR, 2012). As a principle, participation is expected to guide duty bearers (i.e., governments) in their implementation of human rights. Specifically, "States should encourage popular participation in all spheres as an important factor in development and in the full realization of all human rights" (OHCHR, 2012). Emphasis is given to ensuring that all subpopulations, in particular vulnerable and marginalized groups, have the opportunity to actively participate. As such, health system governance should include ensuring platforms for community participation in the design, implementation and monitoring and evaluation of national health strategies (Potts, 2010).

In relation to social participation, the State has the responsibility for creating spaces and conditions of participation to allow vulnerable communities to achieve a greater control over the material, social and political determinants of their own welfare (Potts, 2010). Addressing this concern is fundamental and defines an important part of what the orientation of policy action on health equity will be. While the need for community empowerment and engagement is widely recognized, the actual process is fraught with challenges. Whilst such strategies often start from simple information provision or participation, they do not always culminate in true community collaboration and action. Enabling true community control is also problematic when health agendas or the objectives of a programme have been set externally.

In the process of reviewing how health programmes can better incorporate participatory approaches, it is useful to consider the following questions:

- What is the desired type of participation and which function would it serve, and from whose perspective?

- Have women and men participated equally – both as beneficiaries and as programme staff members? Has the programme considered how gender and other sociocultural norms may impede the participation of women or men and addressed them appropriately?

- What is the level or extent of participation (e.g. from informing to empowering)?

- In which phases of the programme cycle does participation take place (e.g. needs assessment, planning, implementation, monitoring and evaluation) and at which levels (local, district/state, national)?

- How are participatory approaches applied in daily work, and how do they relate to the roles of health personnel?

- Who from within the target population has opportunities to participate (i.e. is there equitable opportunity)?

- What are the mechanisms and resources required by the programme for supporting social participation?

- Beyond the programme, how is social participation supported across the health system and beyond?

Some of these questions are explored in greater detail in this step.

Types and functions of participation: There are many conceptualizations and models for considering the types and functions of participation. Table 6.2 illustrates the functions that different types of participation can have. In designing participatory approaches, it is critical for health authorities to have a clear understanding of the desired function. Otherwise efforts may not have the intended effect. In keeping with participation in the context of a HRBA,

this function should be as "transformative" as possible (see last row), with both the precursor and the end goal for participation (by both the interested health programme managers and the population engaged) being empowerment. Towards empowerment, transformative participation's main function is to "build political capability, critical consciousness and confidence, to enable people and demand rights, and to enhance accountability".

Table 6.2 **Types and functions of participation**

Type of participation	Main function of type of participation	Interest of the health or programme	Interest of the population
Nominal or functional	To enlist people in projects or processes, so as to secure compliance, minimize dissent, lend legitimacy	Legitimation	Inclusion
Instrumental	To make projects or interventions run more efficiently, by enlisting contributions, delegating responsibilities	Efficiency	Cost reduction through access benefits
Representative	To get in tune with public views and values, to garner good ideas, to defuse opposition, to enhance responsiveness	Sustainability and information	Influence and accountability
Transformative	To build political capabilities, critical consciousness and confidence; to enable people to demand rights; to enhance accountability	Empowerment	Empowerment

Sources: Adapted from Villalba Egiluz (2008:301); based on White, 1996; and Gaventa & Cornwall, 2001.

As mentioned, the aim of the "transformative" function is to result in empowerment. "Empowerment" is a debated term with many definitions (Ibrahim & Alkire, 2007). A frequently used definition is "the expansion of assets and capabilities of poor people to participate in, negotiate with, influence, control and hold accountable institutions that affect their lives" (Narayan, 2005).

In this definition and others, two distinct elements emerge. One is related to agency[1] (influenced by people's assets and capabilities) and the second relates to the institutional environment (which offers

people opportunities to exert agency) (Narayan, 2005). In designing participatory approaches, health authorities can be aware of these two distinct elements as well as their linked and reinforcing nature. Acknowledgement of these two distinct elements is in keeping with a HRBA to health (WHO & OHCHR, 2001), which emphasizes among other things:

• Empowering people to know and claim their rights;

• Increasing the ability and accountability of individuals and institutions who are responsible for respecting, protecting and fulfilling rights.

Levels of participation: Various classifications of levels of participation exist; one classification uses a scale from informing, to consulting, to involving, to collaborating, to responsibility in decision-

---

[1] Amartya Sen, in his development of the capability approach, describes agency as "what a person is free to do and achieve in pursuit of whatever goals or values her or she regards as important" (Sen, 1985). This definition links agency to the ability to participate in economic, social and political actions.

making (IAP2, 2007). Independent of how the levels of participation are classified, it is important to acknowledge that each level corresponds to a different set of activities.

Applying a participatory approach across the programme cycle: Likewise, in practice, the levels of participation may vary across a programme's cycle. For instance, across the phases of needs assessment and planning, implementation, monitoring and evaluation, the levels may differ. There may be some phases where, for example, the level of social participation is more towards "informing", and others where it is more towards "collaboration". Health authorities should however, in keeping with a HRBA to participation, consider how to enhance the levels across the programme cycle.

Incorporating platforms and mechanisms for social participation requires resource allocation, both financial and human, as well as supportive programmatic and policy frameworks. This is especially the case if social participation becomes an integral and ongoing/long-term component of the programme's way of working.

Equitable opportunities for participation: It is important to consider *who* is participating, and if the established platforms for participation actually unintentionally exclude anyone. Subpopulations who have lower levels of education and/or are illiterate, live in remote/hard-to-reach areas, have lesser information technology connectivity, are very occupied in meeting basic survival needs and face other adverse daily living conditions, may experience more challenges in participating, even if platforms for this do exist. Likewise, there may be gender norms, roles and relations that introduce power dynamics and/or limit opportunities for engagement in participatory platforms. Particularly when considering social participation as a means for reducing health inequities, health authorities can actively look to promote opportunities for equitable participation by designing mechanisms and platforms that are accessible and appropriate for more marginalized subpopulations and take into account their daily living conditions and cultural and gender norms.

Step 6 Additional reading and resources

Adelaide Statement on Health in All Policies. WHO, Government of South Australia, Adelaide 2010. Available: http://www.who.int/social_determinants/publications/isa/hiap_statement_who_sa_final.pdf?ua=1 (accessed 25 February 2016).

Potts H (2010). Participation and the right to the highest attainable standard of health. Human Rights Centre: University of Essex. Available: http://repository.essex.ac.uk/9714/1/participation-right-highest-attainable-standard-health.pdf (accessed 26 February 2016).

WHO (2014b). Demonstrating a health in all policies analytic framework for learning from experiences: based on literature reviews from Africa, South-East Asia and the Western Pacific. Geneva: World Health Organization. Available: http://apps.who.int/iris/bitstream/10665/104083/1/9789241506274_eng.pdf (accessed 26 February 2016).

WHO (2014c). Social Determinants of Health (website) – Social participation. Available: http://www.who.int/social_determinants/thecommission/countrywork/within/socialparticipation/en/ (accessed 1 March 2016).

CASE STUDY EXAMPLES OF STEP 6 FROM COUNTRY PROGRAMME APPLICATIONS

Chile's Red Tide programme

Chile's national programme for the Control and Prevention of Intoxication by Harmful Algal Blooms, or Red Tide, one of the six programmes that participated in the review and redesign initiative in 2009/2010, is an environmental health programme that aims to prevent morbidity and mortality due to respiratory paralysis, derived from the consumption of contaminated shellfish. The component interventions, implemented nationally and by regional and local Red Tide committees, include: monitoring of harvesting areas; education and information; and control-surveillance of product prior to consumption (see the yellow boxes in Figure 6.2).

Upon detection of toxins above permitted levels, the health authorities ban the extraction and sale of shellfish from the affected areas. Overall, the programme was considered successful because no deaths due to algal toxins had been registered for years, although gastroenteritis cases – possibly related to cancer – were registered in official statistics.

From an equity perspective, the review team found that the programme measures generally offered equal protection for all, although some subpopulations, living in remote areas were not covered by environmental monitoring or obtaining adequate information. However, the closure of fishing areas had socioeconomic impacts on artisan shore collectors and divers, who lost their livelihood each time the measure was decreed by the Ministry of Health. The living conditions of the Kawéskar (Alacalufe) indigenous people subsisting almost exclusively on shellfish harvesting were especially affected.

This analysis revealed the contextual interactions of the programme interventions and their impacts on different subpopulations.

STEP 6

Figure 6.2 Contextual interactions of the Red Tide programme interventions and their impacts on different subpopulations

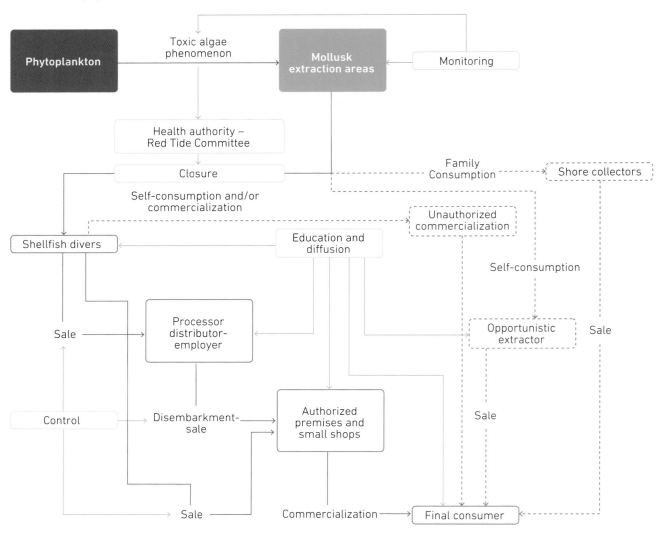

From these emerging findings the review team recognized that the programme needed to:

- Ensure equity of access to environmental monitoring and adequate information (culturally pertinent and translated into indigenous languages); and

- Consider the socioeconomic impacts of its interventions, especially the prohibition of extraction that generated unemployment, rejection and clandestine activities by affected subpopulations.

Source: Ministerio de Salud, Chile, 2010; Solar, 2014.

Proposal of action with other sectors

The conclusion was that the health sector had a responsibility not only for the health outcomes of the programme but also in fostering intersectoral action and social participation to address the socioeconomic impacts of the interventions. This meant deepening collaboration with other sectors such as the National Fishing Service, the Ministry of Labour and the Ministry of Social Development by integrating them in the Red Tide committees, together with community representatives, to develop mitigation plans.

Nepal's national adolescent sexual and reproductive health programme

In 2015, a programme review was conducted to ascertain how the national adolescent sexual and reproductive health (ASRH) programme of Nepal could better address equity, gender, human rights and social determinants of health, hence working to ensure that "no adolescent is left behind". The review was led by the Family Health Division of the Ministry of Health and Population Nepal, with support from the WHO and Health Research and Social Development Forum (HERD) and in conjunction with other members of an interdisciplinary review team. The ASRH programme sits within a broader adolescent health and development strategy.

The national ASRH programme was designed to reach all adolescents. However, due to various factors like budget constraints and lack of human resources, many adolescent subpopulations are still deprived of adolescent friendly services. The majority of young people live in rural areas. The age-specific fertility rate among women 15–19 years in rural populations is twice that of urban. But at present adolescent friendly services are mainly concentrated in well-equipped health facilities in easily accessible areas.

Following its completion of the analysis on "subpopulations being missed by the programme or who benefit less", the review team identified "rural hard-to-reach" subpopulations for further analysis across the subsequent steps of the review, but other groups such as urban slum residents and ethnic minorities were also considered important and also intersect with this subpopulation. Social participation of these adolescents in all stages of programme planning, implementation, monitoring and evaluation was considered to be a critical element for improving the programme overall and for greater equity and attention to gender and human rights issues.

Proposal of actions to foster social participation in the programme

Social participation was considered by the review team as important since it increases community ownership of the programme and makes it accountable to the target population. The ASRH programme has insured the social participation by involving various stakeholders, such as school teachers, local social workers and leaders, and adolescents, in local health forum committees. However, involving adolescent representatives is not mandatory according to the ASRH programme implementation guideline (2011) and their inclusion as invitee members of the local health forum committees is optional. The review team considered that in addition to the full participation of adolescents of both sexes in these committees, other mechanisms should involve adolescents and youths in all of the activities related to ASRH.

In order to address equity, gender, human rights and social determinants of health in the ASRH programme, the following mechanisms for strengthening participation were proposed by the review team:

- Adolescents should be full members of local health forum committees at local level (with one male and one female youth member).

- Formation, coordination and mobilization of child clubs, junior and youth Red Cross circles.

- Ensure meaningful participation of society leaders and adolescents in each step of the programme (design, implementation, monitoring and evaluation).

- Make necessary changes in guidelines and protocols to ensure the participation of all concerned stakeholders.

- Conduct advocacy to sensitize the community about the importance of ASRH.

The review team identified some of the facilitating and hindering factors for furthering social participation in relation to ASRH, which these proposals would address (see Table 6.3).

STEP 6

Table 6.3 Facilitating and hindering factors for social participation

Facilitating factors	Hindering factors
Ward citizen forum exists in each district	ASRH is perceived as less important
Social mobilizers in each district engaged in local decision-making bodies	Inadequate empowerment of adolescents to exercise their rights and duties
Child clubs, Junior Red Cross etc.	Negative perception about ASRH issues in society
Adolescents are invitees in different bodies such as health forum committees	

Source: Ministry of Health and Population, Nepal, 2016.

STEP 6 ACTIVITIES SUMMARY

Table 6.4 contains the activities that the review team will develop to finalize Step 6. It also indicates the questions that orient the activities and the methods used.

Table 6.4 Summary of activities to develop Step 6: Consider intersectoral action and social participation as central elements

Questions	Activity components	Methods
Activity 1: Identify and characterize intersectoral action in the key stages of the programme		
What sectors are relevant for the outcome of the programme? Which are most relevant? What is their engagement with the health sector and programme?	• Identify sectors relevant to the key stages of the programme and prioritize three sectors. • Identify the type of relationship the health sector develops with these sectors. • Identify facilitating factors and obstacles for intersectoral action.	Review team reflection Analysis of additional data sources Review team discussion
Activity 2: Prioritize and develop/improve intersectoral action in the key stages of the programme		
What sectors are most relevant in each key stage to address identified barriers and inequities in health? What actions or interventions of other sectors are necessary to address identified barriers and inequities in health?	• Analyse the main motivations, mechanisms and models behind the health sector to develop intersectoral action for the sectors identified. • Identify some specific recommendations and ways that the health sector and other sectors prioritized can facilitate. • Suggest ways to communicate to other sectors the need for engagement.	Review team reflection Evidence review and data analysis Data analysis and interpretation Review team deliberation
Activity 3: Describe the current approach to social participation by the programme		
In which stages of the programme is there the opportunity for social participation? What is the motivation or purpose of this from the health programme's perspective?	• Describe the types of social participation currently applied by the programme. • Identify facilitating factors and obstacles for social participation, including gender and other sociocultural factors. • Identify the ways in which the programme currently incorporates social participation across the programme cycle. • Identify how the programme currently provides opportunities for equitable participation.	Review team reflection Evidence review and data analysis
Activity 4: Prioritize and develop/improve actions for social participation in key stages of the programme that contribute to addressing the barriers and facilitating factors		
What recommendations should be made with regard to enhancing social participation?	• Develop specific recommendations and propose mechanisms to enhance social participation in the programme. • Suggest ways to communicate to stakeholders the crucial role of social participation.	Review team reflection

STEP 6

STEP 6 ACTIVITY GUIDE

The primary focus of these exercises for Step 6 entails discussion and reflection by the review team to consider the role of intersectoral action and social participation as central elements for each key stage of the programme in order to tackle the access barriers and health inequities identified. The review team will identify interventions or activities to carry out with these sectors and community and civil society stakeholders. The review team should draw from their own knowledge and experience and can review the checklist findings and, as feasible and relevant in the training context and in the follow-up time allocated for working on the exercises, review additional programme documents and available data sources.

INTERSECTORAL WORK

ACTIVITY 1

Identify and characterize intersectoral action in the key stages of the programme

Based on the combined knowledge and experiences of the review team members, **which sectors can or cannot influence the outcome of the programme because of their high or low level of interest and influence?**

1.a. To complete this task, the review team can refer to questiotn 11 in the checklist, corresponding to intersectoral work; the other sector(s) and stakeholder(s) identified in Step 5; and those relevant to the barriers and facilitating factors identified in Step 4. The review team should then put their answers in the following table.

Name of sector or stakeholder	Influence/power over the outcome of the programme (high or low)	Interest/stake in issue (high or low)	Likely position in relation to the programme (positive, negative, conflict)	Engages in what stage of the programme
1.				
2.				
3.				
4.				
5.				
6.				
7.				
8.				
9.				
10.				

Source: Adapted from: Module 7: The role of non-government stakeholders in HiAP/whole-of-society approaches (WHO, 2015:93–108).

1.b. Based on the combined knowledge and experiences of the review team members, **what type of relationship is developed by the health sector or programme with other sectors?** Using the following table, please indicate one key type of relationship for each sector.

Type of relationship of health sector with other sectors	Education	Social planning	Social protection	Women's affairs	Labour	Housing	Agriculture	Financing	Other sector(s) as relevant
Information									
Cooperation									
Coordination									
Integration									

1.c. Explain your answer here in one to two sentences per sector.

1.d. Identify the three sectors that have potential to have the greatest impact on programme outcomes, contributing to overcoming barriers and decreasing inequities on the basis of the first table in this activity (asking about level of influences).

CONSIDER INTERSECTORAL ACTION AND SOCIAL PARTICIPATION AS CENTRAL ELEMENTS
STEP 6

1.e. In your experience, what are the main facilitating factors for carrying out intersectoral work [with _____ sector] in relation to the programme? Complete this exercise for each of the three sectors prioritized in the previous exercise.

1.f. In your experience, what are the main obstacles to carrying out intersectoral work [with _____ sector] in relation to the programme? Look back at the answers in the checklist on challenges, and see if the team has anything to add. Complete this exercise for each of the three sectors prioritized.

ACTIVITY 2

Prioritize and develop/improve intersectoral action in the key stages of the programme

In the previous activity, the review team identified three sectors with which enhanced collaboration would be beneficial. It is now relevant to better understand the way in which the programme has worked so far with other sectors. If intersectoral actions are carried out, the review team should aim to delineate the main motivations, mechanisms and models behind the engagement with the other sector. The following table helps in that sense.

2.a. This table should be completed for the three main sectors that the review team has prioritized.

Describe the sector analysed			
Questions	Area	Tick	Describe briefly
What is the purpose or objective of working together?	To reach a wider coverage		
	To consult on the definition of policies or regulations		
	To launch a campaign		
	To solve a particular matter/issues		
	To undertake joint planning in order to achieve shared goals		
	Other (provide details)		
What is shared?	Share and exchange information		
	Share activities and resources*		
	Share power and capabilities*		
	Share authority*		

STEP 6

Describe the sector analysed			
Questions	Area	Tick	Describe briefly
When and how is intersectoral work carried out?	Intersectoral work is incidental or reactive to a problem or situation		
	Intersectoral work is mainly to support programme implementation		
	Working together includes formulation, implementation and evaluation, but only for specific moments or instances. For example, there is joint planning that results in plans and budgets for each sector, although there is no single plan that integrates all sectors		
	Working together encompasses the whole policy cycle of formulation, implementation and evaluation of work through the whole policy cycle with high-level political mandates, support structures and guidelines integrating all sectors		

* Source: Adapted from Bryson et al, 2006.

Based on the combined knowledge and experiences of the review team members, please answer the following question.

2.b. What actions or interventions of other sectors are necessary to address identified barriers and inequities in health? Complete this exercise for each of the three sectors prioritized.

Identified sector (other than health sector)	What is specifically recommended to be done by the other sector?	What should the health sector do to enable/facilitate this?
	1.	
	2.	
	3.	
	4.	

2.c. Now consider communication and advocacy with other sectors to build the level of engagement desired.
For each of the three prioritized sectors, write a paragraph for each sector setting out the arguments the team would use to convince them to engage.

SOCIAL PARTICIPATION

ACTIVITY 3

Describe the current approach to social participation by the programme

Based on the combined knowledge and experiences of the review team members, please answer the following questions.

3.a. In which stages of the programme is there currently social participation?

3.b. What is the motivation or purpose of this participation from the health programme's perspective? Indicate the type of social participation applied in the different key stages of the programme and explain. Please see Table 6.2 in the background reading for explanations of the types of participation.

Key stage of programme	Type of social participation			
	Legitimation	Efficiency	Sustainability and information	Empowerment

3.c. In which ways does the programme now incorporate social participation into the general programme cycle, i.e. the needs assessment, planning, implementation, and monitoring and evaluation of the programme?

Programme cycle component	Ways in which social participation is currently incorporated	How does the review team think that this can be improved?
Needs assessment		
Planning		
Implementation		
Monitoring and evaluation		

3.d. If the programme now incorporates social participation, how does it take specific measures to ensure equitable opportunities for participation by women and men from different subpopulations? For instance, which efforts are made to ensure that participation is feasible for rural, remote, poor and illiterate subpopulations, not only for more affluent, literate and urban populations? Has the programme considered how gender and other sociocultural norms may impede social participation and has the programme addressed these appropriately?

3.e. Based on the combined knowledge and experiences of the review team members, what are the main facilitating factors for ensuring social participation?

3.f. Based on the combined knowledge and experiences of the review team members, what are the main obstacles to carrying out social participation work in relation of the programme? Refer back to the checklist work already done on this and expand. Think also of social participation of the prioritized subpopulation when responding to this question.

STEP 6

ACTIVITY 4

Prioritize and develop/improve actions for social participation in key stages of the programme that contribute to addressing the barriers and facilitating factors

4.a. For each key stage of the programme and in relation to the prioritized subpopulation discuss: **What mechanisms, actions or recommendations should be made with regard to enhancing social participation (i.e. acknowledging that participation is both a fundamental human right and that it is leverage through which to work towards leaving no one behind)?**

Specific action or recommendation for the inclusion of social participation in the redesign of the health programme	What would the health sector need to do to make this happen?

4.b. Now consider how to communicate to stakeholders the crucial role of social participation. Please produce a paragraph with the argument to communicate this proposal.

STEP 6 OUTPUTS

Congratulations, the review team has completed the analysis for Step 6!

The review team should **summarize the outputs of Step 6 in a short report (approximately two to five pages)**, while this analysis is fresh in your minds. The output summary should clearly and succinctly capture the main findings and decisions of the review team across the activities in this step. You will be using these output summaries from across the steps towards the end of the review process in Step 7 to "bring it all together" in considering redesign options and for a final review team report on the review process.

The output summary for Step 6 should cover the following components:

• Description of the intersectoral action taking place in the programme currently (including which sectors, the type of relationship, and the main motivations, mechanisms and models behind this engagement and other details).

• Description of the main challenges and facilitating factors for intersectoral action in relation to the programme.

• Outline of the review team's proposals/ recommendations for developing or improving

intersectoral action with specific sectors in key stages of the programme to address the identified barriers and inequities in health, including what the health sectors should do and how to build the policy discourse with these sectors.

• Description of the social participation taking place in the programme currently for each critical key stage (including which with stakeholders, for what motivations or purpose, and the type of participation) and how the programme incorporates social participation into the general programme cycle and any specific measures to ensure equitable opportunities for participation.

• Description of the main challenges and facilitating factors for social participation in the programme.

• Outline of the review team's proposals/ recommendations for enhancing social participation in the programme to address the identified barriers and facilitators, including through which mechanisms or actions, with which stakeholders, what the health sectors should do and how to communicate with them.

REFERENCES

Adelaide Statement on Health in All Policies. WHO, Government of South Australia, Adelaide 2010. Available: http://www.who.int/social_determinants/publications/isa/hiap_statement_who_sa_final.pdf?ua=1 (accessed 25 February 2016).

Bryson JM, Crosby BC, Stone MM (2006). The design and implementation of cross-sector collaborations: Propositions from the literature. Public Administration Review. 2006:66(s1);44–55.

CSDH (2008). Closing the gap in a generation: Health equity through action on the social determinants of health. Final Report of the Commission on Social Determinants of Health. Geneva: World Health Organization. Available: http://whqlibdoc.who.int/publications/2008/9789241563703_eng.pdf (accessed 25 February 2016).

Drèze J, Sen AK (1989). Hunger and Public Action. Oxford, UK: Clarendon Paperbacks, Oxford University Press.

Gaventa J, Cornwall A (2001). Power and Knowledge. In: Reason P, Bradbury H, eds. Handbook of Action Research: Participative. Inquiry and Practice. London: Sage Publications. Available: http://www.alastairmcintosh.com/general/verene/Gaventa%20and%20Cornwall%20on%20Power.pdf (accessed 25 February 2016).

IAP2 (2007). International Association of Public Participation 2 – Spectrum of Public Participation. Available: http://c.ymcdn.com/sites/www.iap2.org/resource/resmgr/imported/IAP2%20Spectrum_vertical.pdf (accessed 25 February 2016).

Ibrahim S, Alkire S (2007). Agency and Empowerment: A proposal for internationally comparable indicators. OPHI Working Paper Series. Available: http://www.ophi.org.uk/wp-content/uploads/OPHI-wp04.pdf (accessed 25 February 2016).

STEP 6

International Health Conference (1946). Constitution of the World Health Organization as adopted by the International Health Conference, New York, 19–22 June 1946; signed on 22 July 1946 by the representatives of 61 States (Official Records of the World Health Organization) and entered into force on 7 April 1948.

Kickbusch I, Buckett K (2010). Implementing Health in All Policies. Adelaide 2010. Department of Health. Government of South Australia. Available: http://www.who.int/sdhconference/resources/implementinghiapadel-sahealth-100622.pdf (accessed 25 February 2016).

Ministry of Health and Population, Nepal (2016). Review of the national ASRH programme to address equity, social determinants of health, gender and human rights. Final report prepared by Health Research and Social Development Forum (HERD).

Ministerio de Salud (2010). Documento Tectinco I, II, III: Serie de Documentos Técnicos del Rediseño de los Programas desde la Perspectiva de Equidad y Determinantes Sociales. Subsecretaría de Salud Pública: Santiago. [Ministry of Health, Chile (2010). Technical documents I, II, and III for supporting the review and redesign of public health programmes from the perspective of equity and social determinants of health. Santiago: Undersecretary for Public Health.] Materials in Spanish only.

Narayan D (2005). Measuring empowerment: Cross-disciplinary perspectives. Washington, DC: The World Bank. Available: https://openknowledge.worldbank.org/bitstream/handle/10986/7441/344100PAPER0Me101Official0use0only1.pdf?sequence=1 (accessed 25 February 2016).

OHCHR (2012). United Nations Declaration on the Right to Development. Geneva. Available: http://www.ipu.org/splz-e/unga14/rtd.pdf (accessed 25 February 2016).

Potts H (2010). Participation and the right to the highest attainable standard of health. Human Rights Centre: University of Essex. Available: http://repository.essex.ac.uk/9714/1/participation-right-highest-attainable-standard-health.pdf (accessed 26 February 2016).

Sen AK (1985). Well-being, agency and freedom. The Dewey Lectures 1984. Journal of Philosophy. 1985;82(4):169-221.

Solar O (2014). Presentation overview of the review and redesign process. WHO meeting in Alicante, Spain. June 2014.

Solar O, Cunill N (2015). Intersectorialidad y equidad en salud en América Latina: una aproximación analítica. Programa Especial de Desarrollo Sostenible y Equidad en Salud. OPS. Washington, DC: OPS/OMS.

Solar O, Irwin A (2010). A conceptual framework for action on the social determinants of health. Social Determinants of Health Discussion Paper 2 (Policy and Practice). Geneva: World Health Organization. Available: http://www.who.int/sdhconference/resources/ConceptualframeworkforactiononSDH_eng.pdf (accessed 26 February 2016).

Solar O, Valentine N, Albrech D, Rice M (2009). Moving forward to equity in health: What kind of intersectoral action is needed? An approach to an intersectoral typology. In: 7th Global Conference for Health Promotion, Nairobi, Kenya.

Villalba Egiluz U (2008). El empoderamiento entre la participación en el desarrollo y la economía social. In: Espinosa, B, ed. Mundos del Trabajo, Pluralidad y Transformaciones Contemporáneas. Quito: FLACSO-Ecuador, Ministerio de Cultura. Available: http://www.flacsoandes.edu.ec/biblio/catalog/resGet.php?resId=16753 (accessed 26 February 2016).

White S (1996). Depoliticising development: the uses and abuses of participation. Development in practice. 1996;6(1)6–15.

World Conference on Social Determinants of Health (2011). Rio Political Declaration on Social Determinants of Health. Rio de Janeiro. Available: http://www.who.int/sdhconference/declaration/Rio_political_declaration.pdf?ua=1 (accessed 26 February 2016).

World Health Assembly (2014). Resolution WHA67.12. Contributing to social and economic development: sustainable action across sectors to improve health and health equity). Geneva: World Health Organization. Available: http://apps.who.int/gb/ebwha/pdf_files/WHA67/A67_R12-en.pdf (accessed 26 February 2016).

WHO (1986). Ottawa Charter for Health Promotion. Geneva: World Health Organization.

WHO (2008). Health equity through intersectoral action. An analysis of 18 country case studies. Geneva: World Health Organization. Available: http://www.who.int/social_determinants/resources/health_equity_isa_2008_en.pdf (accessed 26 February 2016).

WHO (2013). The 8th Global Conference on Health Promotion. Helsinki statement on Health in All Policies. Geneva: World Health Organization. Available: http://www.who.int/healthpromotion/conferences/8gchp/8gchp_helsinki_statement.pdf (accessed 26 February 2016).

WHO (2014a). Burden of disease from Household Air Pollution for 2012. Summary of results. Available: http://www.who.int/phe/health_topics/outdoorair/databases/FINAL_HAP_AAP_BoD_24March2014.pdf (accessed 26 February 2016).

WHO (2014b). Demonstrating a health in all policies analytic framework for learning from experiences: based on literature reviews from Africa, South-East Asia and the Western Pacific. Geneva: World Health Organization. Available: http://apps.who.int/iris/bitstream/10665/104083/1/9789241506274_eng.pdf (accessed 26 February 2016).

WHO (2014c). Social Determinants of Health (website) – Social participation. Available: http://www.who.int/social_determinants/thecommission/countrywork/within/socialparticipation/en/ (accessed 1 March 2016).

WHO (2015). Health in All Policies: Training Manual. Geneva: World Health Organization.

WHO and OHCHR (2001). Factsheet No. 31. The Right to Health. Geneva: World Health Organization. Available: http://www.who.int/hhr/activities/Right_to_Health_factsheet31.pdf (accessed 26 February 2016).

WHO Regional Office for Europe (1978). Declaration of Alma-Ata. Available: http://www.euro.who.int/__data/assets/pdf_file/0009/113877/E93944.pdf (accessed 26 February 2016).

Step7

Produce a redesign proposal to act on the review findings

Overview

The redesign step is the most critical and creative part of the Innov8 approach. In this step, the review team consolidates the learning and analysis from the previous steps and considers how this can be applied to changing the programme to become more responsive to equity, gender, human rights and social determinants of health. The review team then produces a proposal that delineates what is to be done, at what level, how it should be done and who should be involved.

Step 7 activities guide the review team members to produce a new programme theory, which incorporates the theory of inequities from the previous step, and is more equity enhancing and gender responsive and rights based. This new programme theory and the recommendations from the previous steps orient the changes and adjustments that constitutes the redesign proposal of the programme.

The five activities of Step 7 are:

1) Developing a new programme theory that is equity enhancing and gender responsive and rights based;

2) Identifying the scope and level (national, regional, local) of the proposed changes;

3) Finalizing the revised diagram and theory of the programme to be more equity enhancing and gender responsive and rights based;

4) Delineating a short-term plan for the implementation of the proposed programme adjustments and redesign; and

5) Producing a report with the redesign proposal.

During this step, the review team complements its experience and knowledge of the programme with additional evidence on the effectiveness and feasibility of potential new interventions or adjustments to the programme. Step 7 may imply additional actions, such as possibly conducting feasibility studies and pilots, and integration into programme planning that must be approached in accordance with the programmatic and national context. Moving towards implementation is very specific to the national and programme context, as well as resource constraints. Hence, providing comprehensive guidance on all aspects is beyond the scope of this handbook.

The main output of Step 7 is the report detailing the proposal for redesign of the programme, including a **new programme theory** and **new logic model diagram** of the revised programme. This report is also the main outcome of fully applying the Innov8 approach outlined in this handbook. It is used to further consult with stakeholders and develop the proposed programme changes towards implementation. This report will also contain an output from the next chapter (Step 8) – the plan to monitor and evaluate the revised programme.

Objectives of Step 7

> Propose a new programme theory that addresses the theory of inequities, defining the priorities and objectives for redesign.

> Identify the level (national, regional, local) and scope of the proposed changes.

> Consider implementation aspects to further the proposal, including pilots and other studies.

> Produce a report with the redesign proposal of the programme.

PRODUCE A REDESIGN PROPOSAL TO ACT ON THE REVIEW FINDINGS
STEP 7

BACKGROUND READING FOR STEP 7

This reading provides a basic orientation for considering how to redesign the programme to strengthen equity, gender, human rights and social determinants of health perspectives and looks at:

- The components of the redesign phase;
- The added value of realist evaluation for programme review and redesign;
- Reviewing the evidence base;
- Priority setting;
- The scope and level of change;
- Engagement with other health sector actors, other sectors and civil society; and
- Moving from a proposal towards actual programme changes.

The components of the redesign phase

In the redesign phase, the review team should consider the modifications that could be undertaken, identifying the applicable programme areas/functions and level of the action (national, regional or local). The agreement about the changes to the programme constitutes the proposal for redesign. The proposal for redesign also presents an initial implementation plan, addressing how, in which timeframe, with what resources and under whose responsibility the proposed changes would be further advanced (in terms of considering their feasibility, piloting, learning lessons and scaling up).

The process of producing a redesign proposal, and potentially piloting it, may include the following components:

- Identify objectives and priorities for redesign based on the theory of inequities developed in the previous step;

- Review of the evidence base for interventions/ adjustments that can promote the right to health and address social determinants and barriers associated with health inequity;

- Consider how to address gender norms, roles and relations for women and men and their impact on access to and control over resources;

- Identify the scope and level of changes (national, regional, local);

- Engage with other health sector actors (beyond the health programme), as well as other sectors and civil society, about the potential changes to the programme; and

- Mechanisms, such as pilots, to test and refine the proposed changes to the programme, before scaling up.

Figure 7.1. Components of producing the redesign proposal

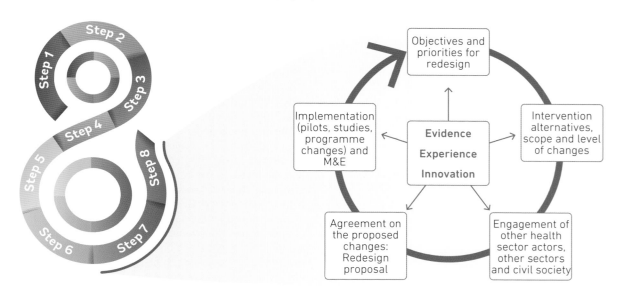

The activities in the redesign step should be aligned with the programme planning and review cycle to enable the integration and sustainability of the potential changes.

The value-added of realist evaluation for programme review and redesign

As emphasized previously, realist evaluation is the basis of the Innov8 methodology, focusing on "what works for whom in what circumstances and in what respects, and how?" (Pawson & Tilley, 1997; Pawson & Tilley 2004). It emphasizes: (i) identifying the mechanisms that produce observable programme effects; and (ii) testing these mechanisms and other context variables that have impacts on the observed effects (Pawson & Tilley, 2004). It also recognizes the complexity of the transformation processes sought by health programmes and interventions aimed at leaving no one behind, and the importance of context and of other sectoral influences (Dunn et al, 2013).

Following this approach, the application of Innov8 aims to shed light on how and why a programme:

• Is more useful and effective for some populations than others;

• Encounters specific barriers for some populations;

• Can have unintended consequences or not;

• Does or does not work depending on certain conditions and contextual influences; and

• May generate unintended inequities because certain activities are not present or change the contextual factors.

The knowledge generated in the previous steps should enable the review team to recommend changes in the health programme, accounting for the complexity in its analysis and redesign proposal. This is a challenging, but essential task in unlocking entry points to act to redress the issues of equity, gender, human rights and social determinants. By applying realist evaluation thinking to health programmes, the review and redesign methodology aims to build this capacity.

PRODUCE A REDESIGN PROPOSAL TO ACT ON THE REVIEW FINDINGS
STEP 7

Reviewing the evidence base

The redesign phase aims to deepen the knowledge of the review team on how to maximize the functioning of the programme for different subpopulations by tackling the causes of the differences in access and the results. Once this is done, it is time to consider the potential changes to the programme. This requires drawing from the evidence base on the:

• Health topic addressed by the programme, particularly focusing on proven interventions with equity-enhancing, gender responsiveness and rights-based potential;

• Adaptations for the reduction of health inequities;

• Innovative, effective approaches to intersectoral action and social participation; and

• Contributions of health programmes to wider health systems strengthening, particularly in the context of reforms towards UHC.

A primary concern is that any adjustments to the programme, while building in equity-oriented interventions, are in keeping with the established best practice evidence base for addressing the programmatic issue at hand. Nevertheless, as Asthana & Halliday (2006) note, the kind of evidence predominant in the published literature may "attenuate public health decisions," (Rychetnik et al, 2002:125, cited in Asthana & Halliday 2006) due to the emphasis on biomedical interventions rather than social and economic policies, the targeting of individuals rather than communities or populations, and the focus on the influence of proximal rather than structural determinants of health. Closely related, is the dissonance between systematic reviews, which focus largely on individual interventions, and types of approaches that would effectively reduce health inequalities, encompassing solutions at different levels to address wider issues, such as the redistributive effects of fiscal policies or economic investment to counter unemployment. In general, there is a paucity of good quality evaluation studies on these more "upstream" interventions, in part because it is easier and more politically acceptable to research "downstream" causes and solutions (Macintyre et al, 2001).

Priority setting

Defining the potential adjustments to the programme is a decision-making process of planning and resource allocation, which necessarily requires establishing priorities. Often the rationale for defining priorities is implicit. In contrast, explicit priority setting tries to spell out criteria focusing on principles, norms and values to guide the decisions (Kenny & Joffres, 2008). Being very clear about the criteria used and the rationale for this is important in order to justify and in due course advocate for the redesign proposal.

Throughout the full review process, at different points the review team has had to establish priorities (for instance, in identifying the relevant subpopulations experiencing inequity, in defining the critical key stages of the programme, and now in this step in establishing priorities for redesign). A brief summary of common criteria employed in different methodologies of prioritization in public health is summarized in Table 7.1.

Table 7.1 Example criteria for prioritization

Criteria to identify priority problems (programmes)	Criteria to identify priority subpopulations	Criteria to prioritize interventions
Conceptualization (promotion, prevention, curative – upstream, downstream determinants)	Epidemiologic (magnitude, frequency)	Health equity impact
Impact (health, social)	Vulnerability (risk)	Effectiveness
Magnitude	Disadvantaged subpopulations (by sex, ethnicity, social class, etc.)	Expertise
Urgency	Social preference	Feasibility
Public and political connotations		Ease in implementation
Availability of solutions		Legal considerations
Cost of acting/not acting		System impacts
Responsibility		Return on investment
Considers gender norms, roles and relations for women and men and how they can affect access to and control over resources		Considers gender norms, roles and relations for women and men and how they can affect access to and control over resources

From the lens of equity, gender, human rights and social determinants, the criteria in Table 7.1 have different weight and coherence. The review team may also want to draw from work on equity and fairness on the path towards UHC (WHO, 2014). As applicable to the types of barriers identified, the review team can consider the "unacceptable trade-offs" described. The review team may also want to consider criteria in relation to gender mainstreaming in health programmes (WHO, 2011).

The scope and level of change

In further considering the design and operational reality of the potential changes to the programme, the review team should clarify the scope of the change and the details of the specific adjustment.

This involves specifying the level of implementation – national, state/province, district or local levels. Some adjustments that are legislative or regulatory in nature may best be made at national levels (for instance, if there is a law that restricts access to certain subpopulations, or the need to regulate actions of another sector like food and agriculture to address key underlying determinants of health). Other adjustments may be more linked to service delivery, or need to respond to specific on-the-ground operational realities, and hence be appropriate for execution at regional/state or local levels.

When deciding on the level of implementation of the proposed changes, keeping in mind how these will account for the heterogeneity of subpopulations is central.

When contemplating the scope of the proposed adjustment, these questions may be useful:

- **Is there a change to the programme contents?** That is, does the proposed change involve incorporation of a new intervention, service, awareness-raising platform, etc.? If so, at what level will it be implemented? If it is national in nature, does its design account for subnational heterogeneity?

- **Are there proposed changes to the structure and organization of the programme that influence**

STEP 7

execution or delivery? Do the proposed adjustments to the programme entail shifts in delivery channels and/or implementation mechanisms? If so, how will subnational variations in programme capacity (and wider health system capacity) influence this?

- **Are there proposed changes to the management processes and financing mechanisms?** Do the proposed adjustments involve changing the ways needs assessments, planning, budgeting, resource allocation, payment of providers, and other management and financing tasks are done? For example, are there specific budget lines for work on gender equality and/or ethnic minority health? Are there new partners (e.g. like other sectors) with which some interventions/activities should be jointly conducted?

- **Are there proposed changes to the human resources?** Do the proposed adjustments entail changes to pre-service or continuing education for health professionals, task-shifting, use of community mediators/volunteers in activities, or changes to human resources policies (e.g. for recruiting and retaining staff in rural areas)? Do the proposed

adjustments involve having both male and female team members at all decision-making levels?

- **Are there proposed improvements to the normative/standard-setting, regulation or legislation work of the programme?** Does the review team foresee the need for revised or new protocols, standards, guidelines or other normative work? Likewise, are changes to regulation or legislation (e.g. regulation of costs for services offered by private sector providers, legislation for population-based interventions involving other sectors) foreseen in order to create a more enabling environment for health equity?

- **Do the changes involve any mechanism to empower the prioritized subpopulation to know and act on their rights and entitlements in relation to the programme?**

- **Do the changes involve ways to identify, address and/or transform harmful gender norms, roles and relations?**

- **Do the changes involve other sectors beyond the health sector to find solutions to health inequities and more effectiveness of the programme?**

Engagement with other health sector actors, other sectors and civil society

Suggesting adjustments to a programme will require consultations with stakeholders in the health sector and beyond to explore feasibility, get buy-in and build partnerships. The processes leading to the proposal for redesign should be participatory and open to discussion and debate. Spaces need to be created where stakeholders from different parts of the programme (at national and subnational levels) can discuss the advantages for both the programme and the subpopulations being considered. To the extent possible, these would be integrated into ongoing existing programme review or implementation-related meetings. Beyond the direct programme being reviewed, it will likely be very important to also liaise with stakeholders in other parts of the health system that are implicated by the proposed adjustments (i.e. that may manage human resource training, retention, deployment; financial protection schemes; essential medicines, etc.). Where other sectors are involved,

the respective authorities also need to be brought to the table.

The review team will likely meet with resistance from some stakeholders. It is likely that a range of doubts or concerns will be expressed by stakeholders in relation to the emerging recommendations derived from the review. Drawing from the countries in which the review methodology has been applied thus far, some examples of these include:

- **Argument I: Resource constraints imply that equity, gender and rights issues can only be addressed once the programme has addressed other needs.** In counter-arguing this, it is important to stress that taking an equity-enhancing and gender and rights responsive approach in programming does not necessarily mean higher costs or more financing for implementation. In fact, these can optimize the use of existing resources by identifying subpopulations not accessing services and prioritizing the use of resources accordingly (grounded in the ideas of progressive/proportionate universalism).[1] This in turn has potential to improve the overall performance of the programme and ultimately overall population health. Emerging evidence has highlighted the benefits of a progressive universalism approach. While further research is required, a modelling study on child survival, health and nutrition shows that an equity-oriented service delivery model will do more than conventional/mainstream approaches to reduce mortality, health inequities and stunting (Carrera et al, 2012).

- **Argument II: The health sector is not in a position to act on wider determinants of health.**
  The counter-argument is that action on the social and environmental determinants of health is a core part of the stewardship function of health systems. The review methodology identifies precise entry points for engaging with other sectors based on real programmatic needs. It evidences how the

---

[1] Prioritization of an equity-oriented approach through what has been called "progressive universalism" will help ensure that marginalized populations benefit at least as much as those who are better off (Gwatkin & Ergo, 2011). Acknowledging the detriments to equity and inefficiencies in targeting *only* the most disadvantaged, the Marmot Review (Marmot et al, 2010) called for actions towards UHC to indeed be universal, but with a scale and intensity that is proportionate to the level of disadvantage.

contribution of another sector could help the health sector reach its programmatic aims.

- **Argument III: Why make changes to a programme that already is achieving (or is striving to achieve) positive results at aggregate level.** It may be perceived that a health programme works well already because it has positive results at aggregate level where it operates and all that is required is to expand its coverage (i.e. to new districts or states) to improve its effectiveness nationally. As stated previously, basing the measurement of achievements on the average outcomes of the programme can conceal significant inequities.

The redesign phase can also involve further liaison with civil society and programme beneficiaries. While they may already be represented on the review team, more exchange with representatives of the subpopulations that would be most impacted by the proposed reorientations is opportune. It is important that monies and human resources are allocated for this purpose (Potts & Hunt, 2008). If this is not done, there are chances that the interventions – despite their good intentions – receive negative backlash from these communities due to the perceived lack of a participatory approach and/or that they are less effective because they did not account for important contextual or social/cultural factors that consultation with the target community would have illuminated (UN, 2008).

Moving from a proposal towards actual programme changes

Once there is initial clarity on the objectives and priorities, the level and scope of proposed changes, operationalizing ways to address the inequities uncovered in the review process will require bold, innovative thinking. A next step can be to conduct feasibility studies or pilots. The former is an analysis of the potential of a proposed project; its main purpose it to determine the technical and financial viability of a proposed change as well as to assist in identifying or clarifying activities, cost, timeframes and/or requirements (Berrie, 2007).

In an ideal scenario, changes to the programme should be piloted on a small scale and for a long enough period to test their efficiency/effectiveness within the context of programme operations before scaling up to national roll-out of the intervention. Piloting allows

for testing implementation plans and identifying weaknesses and oversights, analysing costs associated with the changes or new interventions, assessing any unintended consequences and/or any secondary benefits, ensuring smooth linkages to other components of the programme, and identifying possible barriers and facilitating factors. All of this will provide important insight on how to adapt and scale up the interventions so that they meet the actual intended aims and objectives of redesign.

In Chile, the six programme review teams developed pilots, which were of different types:

- **Pilots designed to enhance or complement the analysis of equity,** in response to the lack of information during the review cycle. The study aimed

PRODUCE A REDESIGN PROPOSAL TO ACT ON THE REVIEW FINDINGS
STEP 7

to help prioritize the programme redesign's focus and level of intervention.

- **Pilots testing intervention alternatives.** During the review process, various potentially feasible interventions were identified for development in the programme redesign. In this case, the pilot was intended to test some of these interventions in order to recommend the most feasible ones with the best short- and medium term results.

- **Pilots designed to test and prove some of the hypotheses proposed in the redesign**

proposal, taking into account the theory underlying the programme's approach to health equity. This pilot sought to provide a more solid knowledge-base and foundation for the design of certain changes proposed in the programme's operations.

- **Pilots implementing the proposed redesign of the programme in a limited geographic area or for a specific social group** in order to evaluate the process, identify associated difficulties and estimate the cost associated with the changes.

Step 7 Additional reading and resources

Evidence based public health tutorial. See: http://phpartners.org/tutorial/04-ebph/index.html (accessed 26 February 2016).

WHO (2014). Making fair choices on the path to universal health coverage. Final report of the WHO Consultative Group on Equity and Universal Health Coverage. Geneva: World Health Organization. Available: http://apps.who.int/iris/

bitstream/10665/112671/1/9789241507158_eng.pdf?ua=1 (accessed 26 February 2016).

WHO (2011). Gender mainstreaming for health managers; a practical approach. Geneva: World Health Organization. Available: http://www.who.int/gender-equity-rights/knowledge/health_managers_guide/en/ (accessed 22 February 2016).

CASE STUDY EXAMPLES OF STEP 7 FROM COUNTRY PROGRAMME APPLICATIONS

Three case studies profiling different aspects of redesign follow. The examples, taken from three different countries, show the scope of potential changes, a revised programme diagram and theory, and example approaches to piloting.

In Nepal, the national adolescent sexual and reproductive health programme was reviewed in late 2015. During the redesign process, the review team developed the exercise highlighting the potential scope of all the changes that could be made (see Table 7.2). Later, these were consulted on more widely and select ones are being advanced at the time of writing.

How the proposed redesign changes are reflected in the revised programme theory is illustrated by the

case of the colorectal cancer screening programme of the Basque Government of Spain, which highlights the specific changes reflected in the new interventions to address barriers, strengthen facilitators and tackle social determinants of health and gender issues in the revised diagram of the key stages of the programme. Also shown is the programme theory developed by the review team in the beginning, contrasted with the revised theory at the end of the redesign process.

Finally, the strategy for moving from a redesign proposal to implementing the proposed changes in the programme may take the form of a pilot implementation, of different types. Two examples from the Chilean experience are presented.

Nepal's national adolescent sexual and reproductive health programme

Table 7.2 Snapshot of the scope of *tentative* redesign proposals for the national adolescent sexual and reproductive health programme, Nepal

Scope of redesign	Tentative redesign proposals
Modification of programme contents (e.g. adapting or introducing services to specifically meet unmet needs in marginalized subpopulations and tackle health determinants)	• Adapt/develop interventions for adolescents in rural hard-to-reach and urbanized slum areas, including out-of-school adolescents, married and migrant adolescents. • Adapt services to account for gender norms, roles, relations that could inhibit seeking services. • If community outreach (beyond using schools) is done by elder providers and adolescents fear lack of confidentiality, adapt for age-sensitivity and privacy, and enhance provider's capacity • Adapt IEC/BCC materials for different needs and target groups and ensure sufficient quantity
Integration with social programmes and other sectors to act on social stratification mechanisms and relevant living/working conditions	• Institutionalize inter- and intrasectoral coordination at national level. • Working through local government to engage other sectors for adolescent health and development, such as to tackle causes of early marriage and pregnancy (e.g. social protection for poor families, education, cultural norms) and the stigma associated with adolescent reproductive health.

Scope of redesign	Tentative redesign proposals
Structural and organizational changes in the way the programme works (e.g. how it coordinates with other sectors, the times and places where services are delivered and by whom)	• Have a **core team** in each of the districts and a **core team** nationally for adolescent health and development that facilitates inter/intrasectoral coordination. • Formation of authorized adolescent health and development committees at different levels (engage Gender Equality and Social Inclusion units at district health offices to ensure coordination of intersectoral activities for disadvantaged youth). • Strengthen the primary health care outreach in rural/remote areas and urban slums also for ASRH (providing training and integration of within their activities) as feasible.

Management and financing improvements (e.g. overcoming barriers to financial protection for specific services)	• Increase investment and assemble evidence on the rationale for investing more in youth (almost one quarter of population), in particular disadvantaged youth.
	• Mainstreaming local resources (and funds) available in other areas.
	• Link up with the Youth Agenda 25 Policy so that resources (funds) can be available through that and advocacy and links with other sectors can be brokered.
	• Improve intra-health sector coordination (through ASRH committee and other) with other programmes that relate to adolescent health, with ideas for this being:
	  – Improve MOH inter-divisional coordination by nominating one person in each division and having a dedicated coordination mechanism;
	  – Use the Adolescent Health and Development Strategy as a platform for supporting coordination, and include focus on disadvantaged populations;
	  – External development partners/Civil Society Organizations align and enhance coordination with equity focus.
	  – Enhance appropriate AFS focus in activities of RH and other health services.

Human resource adjustments (e.g. enabling the availability of adequately skilled staff, as well as their competencies on equity, determinants, gender and human rights issues)	• Enhance the focus on AFS and ASRH in main pre-service and ongoing training opportunities for health professionals and female community health volunteers. • Ensure frontline capacity-building of staff at local health posts in adolescent health, including ASRH, and address staff retention issues through ensured hand-over. • Provide capacity building materials/supports that tackle social and cultural norms that make providers and teachers shy away from ASRH.
Normative/standard-setting, regulation or legislation advancements (e.g. modifications to legislation that may impact the ability of certain subpopulations to access services, or regulation of policies outside of the health sector that influence exposure to risk factors)	• Incorporate into health staff and teacher performance reviews and quality controls measures around ASRH, to correct providers and teachers shying away from ASRH. • Advocate and support to enforce the law against early marriage, including through engaging other sectors and social participation. • Look at standardization criteria for ASRH, to be also equity sensitive for rural remote areas.

Scope of redesign	Tentative redesign proposals
Social participation mechanisms to empower the priority subpopulations	• Adolescent to be member of HFOMC at local level (one male and one female adolescent/youth member). • Strengthen coordination and mobilization of child clubs, junior and youth Red Cross Circles. Form where not present. • Ensure the participation of society leaders and adolescents in each step of the programme (design, implementation, M&E). • Make necessary change in guidelines and protocols to ensure the participation of all concerned stakeholders. • Conduct advocacy to sensitize the community about the importance of adolescent health and development, including ASRH.

Changes to the **ongoing planning, review, monitoring and evaluation cycles** (e.g. inclusion of equity stratifers, equity-oriented targets, and access barriers as a specific agenda item at annual programme review meetings)	• Improving overarching monitoring capacity of programme and capacity to disaggregate data aligned with HMIS.
	• Increase ownership of the programme and appropriate response by the district health system (district management committee, core team idea), and integrate into ASRH into:
	  – District needs assessments.
	  – District planning and budgeting.
	  – M&E (reinforce quality monitoring components, e.g. facility assessment data, and participatory monitoring (social audits).

Redesign proposal for the colorectal cancer screening programme, Basque Government of Spain

The programme redesign included changes in the theory of the programme. On the basis of these, the following changes were proposed for the programme diagram:

• Adjustments to interventions to address important barriers to access in the different key stages and to strengthen facilitating factors;

• New interventions addressing the barriers and social determinants to make the intervention more equity enhancing, gender responsive and rights based.

The revised programme diagram (Figure 7.2), which highlights the adjustments and new activities for the key stages in green, is presented below:

Figure 7.2 Revised programme diagram of the colorectal cancer screening programme

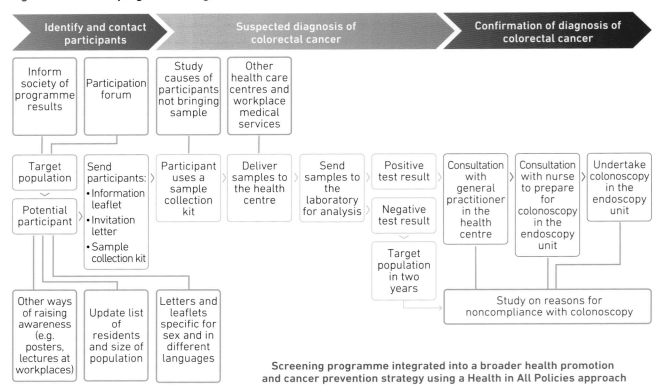

Screening programme integrated into a broader health promotion and cancer prevention strategy using a Health in All Policies approach

Figure 7.3 Comparison of initial and revised programme theories of the colorectal cancer screening programme

STEP 1

Understand the programme theory

- **What it does**
- **What are the expected results of the programme**

> Context
> Heterogeneity
> Mechanism
> Complexity

Initial programme theory

If an informative leaflet and letter are sent to all people aged 50 to 69 years old, inviting them to participate in the colorectal cancer screening programme, they will respond and bring a sample for faecal occult blood testing (FOBT) to the health centre. If the test is positive, they will visit the GP and agree to a colonoscopy. It is also expected that people with a negative result (>92%) will continue participating in the programme when a letter is sent again two years later: they will again collect and deliver another sample for FOBT.

STEP 7

Produce a redesign proposal to act on the review findings

Use the review findings to explore potential adjustments to the programme on the basis of the **theory of inequities**

Revised programme theory

Equitable access to the screening programme will be effective for the whole target population if the different steps take into consideration that not all social groups access in a homogeneous fashion, but rather they demonstrate different behaviour due to socioeconomic conditions and gender. For this reason, just sending an informative leaflet and a letter inviting all people aged 50-69 in the Basque Country to take part in the screening programme will only guarantee a response of approximately 60%. This percentage is liable to vary considerably among the different social groups.

The screening programme needs to be included in a more general strategy of prevention of colorectal cancer and health promotion. Promoting a healthy diet or physical activity requires action across sectors other than health, such as transport, urban planning or regulation of the food industry, as is proposed by the strategy of Health in All Policies (HiAP).

Acting upon the 'determinants of determinants' or upon the 'causes of causes' will allow us to put an end to the underlying causes that influence the different degree of exposure and vulnerability of several social groups facing certain risk factors that contribute to the development of the disease.

PRODUCE A REDESIGN PROPOSAL TO ACT ON THE REVIEW FINDINGS
STEP 7

Piloting redesign proposals – examples from Chile

Table 7.3 Redesign proposal pilots

Programme	Description of the pilot
Oral health	**Implementation in three municipalities with vulnerable populations,** as part of the intersectoral early child development programme, Chile Crece Contigo, with community participation. The priority population is socially vulnerable families, and focuses on the period from pregnancy to the early years of life. This first pilot phase is complementary to qualitative and quantitative studies carried out by the Oral Health Department of the Ministry of Health. The pilot activities aim to improve awareness of the programme and its guarantees and benefits, in order to increase utilization, educate about healthy habits and install opportunities and mechanisms of social participation, such as citizen dialogues.
Cardiovascular health	**Pilot to identify intervention alternatives.** The cardiovascular health programme decided to hold a national call to identify best practices for equity and social determinants at the local level in order to address the needs and circumstances of workers in precarious employment and other groups being left behind. As a result of this call, dozens of innovative interventions were documented, assessed and shared with local programme teams. Additionally, new equity-oriented targets for the priority subpopulation were introduced.

Sources: Ministerio de Salud, Chile, 2010; Ministry of Health and Population, Nepal, 2016; Ministry of Health, Social Services and Equality, Government of Spain, 2012; Portillo et al, 2015; Esnaola, 2015.

STEP 7 ACTIVITIES SUMMARY

Table 7.4 contains the activities and the components of each activity that the review team will develop to develop a redesign proposal.

Table 7.4 Summary of activities to develop Step 7: Produce a redesign proposal to act on the review findings

Questions	Activity components	Methods
Activity 1: Developing a new programme theory that is equity enhancing and gender responsive and rights based		
What are the priorities and objectives for redesign? How should the new programme theory (that addresses equity, social determinants, gender and human rights) be articulated?	• Systematize the emerging findings from the previous review steps. • Identify the objectives and priorities for redesign, exploring how to integrate an explicit commitment to leaving no one behind. • Produce a preliminary new version of the programme theory.	Discussion in the review team, review of findings from the previous steps
Activity 2: Identify the scope and level (national, regional, local) of the proposed changes		
What will be the scope, level and the desired results of the potential programme adjustments? What are necessary changes outside of the health programme?	• Describe the scope and level of the potential programme adjustments. • Consider changes that are needed beyond the direct control of the programme, within and outside the health sector. • Review the desired result of each of the proposed changes.	Discussion in the review team, review of the evidence base, draw from previous activities, consultation with stakeholders
Activity 3: Finalize the revised diagram and theory of the programme to be more equity enhancing and gender responsive and rights based		
What needs to be revised in the programme diagram?	• Revise the programme diagram including the changes (adjustments, new activities) based on the new theory. • Indicate why these changes will produce the expected results.	Discussion in the review team and review of the evidence base
Activity 4: Produce a short-term plan for the implementation of the proposed programme adjustments and redesign		
What implementation details of the proposed programme adjustments should be considered?	• Describe the agreed implementation strategy (pilot, etc.). • Describe the tasks required, responsible parties, required resources and preliminary timeframe.	Discussion in the review team, consultation with stakeholders, draw from previous activities and the evidence
Activity 5: Produce a report with the redesign proposal		
How should the redesign proposal be finalized for presentation?	• Write report of the redesign proposal, following the orientations at the end of the guide.	Compilation by the review team of all previous exercise outputs and drafting of report

STEP 7 ACTIVITY GUIDE

After all of the activities of the review Steps 1–6 are completed, the review team begins work on the redesign phase activities.

ACTIVITY 1

Developing a new programme theory that is equity enhancing and gender responsive and rights based

1.a. Systematize the emerging findings from the Innov8 approach.

The review team should consider the main findings of the review steps to answer the following questions, which seek to summarize the knowledge advanced during the Steps 1–6 and trigger thinking about redesign. The team should document the answers to each question.

- Which are the priority subpopulations (e.g., by sex, age, education level, income, place of residence (rural/urban) and/or other characteristics as appropriate) that need to be better served by the programme in order to leave no one behind?

- Which access barriers are the most important? At what key stage(s) of the programme do they operate? The team should discuss "the most important" barriers in relation to equity, gender and the right to health, and then analyse how the outputs and outcomes of the programme could contribute to these objectives. Was a gender analysis done to highlight the barriers that may be specific to groups of women and men, or boys and girls?

- Which facilitating factors are the most important? At what key stage of the programme do they operate?

- Were programme adjustments to address barriers identified during the review process? If not, make a preliminary proposal for adjustments to address the barriers. An adjustment means proposing a concrete change or a new intervention activity to address the barriers.

- Were programme adjustments to enhance the enabling capacity of facilitating factors identified during the review process? If not, make a preliminary proposal for adjustments to enhance the facilitating factors.

- Which social determinants of health (including gender) and human rights issues were identified as associated with the barriers and which of these are critical in generating the inequities experienced by the priority subpopulation(s)? The key aspect of the question is to identify the adjustments required in the programme activities in order to address the mechanisms generating health inequities.

- What programme adjustments and actions involving other sectors should be included in the redesign, to address the priorities identified during the review? The review team should make a preliminary proposal for adjustments to engage other sectors.

- How could the social participation measures put in place by the programme ensure equitable opportunities for participation (e.g. that the platforms for participation are not inaccessible due to barriers linked to, for example, gender norms, illiteracy or lack of IT connectivity, costs of travel or missed work to participate in meetings, among others)? The review team should make a preliminary proposal for adjustments to enhance social participation.

1.b. Identify the objectives and priorities for redesign.

Taking into account the answers of the previous questions, complete the following table that highlights the priorities for redesign related to different aspects.

	Prioritized sub-population	Prioritized barriers to address	Prioritized intermediary social determinants to address	Prioritized structural social determinants to address	Prioritized sectors for collaboration	Prioritized approaches to social participation
Key programme stage						

Drawing from the above, please indicate the specific objectives for redesign of each programme key stage.

Key programme stage	Specific objectives for redesign

Looking across all specific objectives for redesign of key stages, what would be the summary objective/aim of the redesign?

STEP 7

PRODUCE A REDESIGN PROPOSAL TO ACT ON THE REVIEW FINDINGS
STEP 7

1.c. Produce a preliminary new version of the programme theory.

Drawing from the above, the review team should then consider how the **programme theory** initially developed in Step 2 should be adapted so that the programme can better address equity, gender, human rights and social determinants, summarized in the mechanisms explained in the **theory of inequities of the programme** developed in Step 5. Comparing the programme theory from Step 2 with the theory of inequities of Step 5 will result in reflection on the changes necessary to leave no one behind and achieve greater effectiveness of the programme. Following this reflection, the review team should draft a new programme theory.

In this discussion, the review team should consider the mechanisms of the initial programme theory from Step 2 and those generating inequities in relation to the programme from Step 5. It may be useful to understand that the articulation of a mechanism reflects the reasoning and reactions of collective agents in regard to the resources available in a given context to bring about changes through the implementation of an intervention. These interactions can lead to positive or negative feedback loops (e.g. after negotiation between stakeholders, interference with other interventions), which may or may not lead to the success of the intervention resulting in a change or not (Byng, 2005; Lacouture et al, 2015).

In this respect, the new programme theory should (Lacouture et al, 2015):

- Reflect the embeddedness of the programme within the stratified nature of the social context, where some subpopulations are in more advantaged/privileged positions than others;

- Ensure the programme accounts for barriers and facilitators that subpopulations may face in accessing and benefiting from the programme services;

- Include relevant programmatic activities to address the mechanisms generating the inequities experienced by the subpopulation(s) being missed, which may include actions on intermediary or structural determinants, including through intersectoral action, social participation and enhanced performance and integration within the health sector;

- Be able to respond to the question "if the subpopulation does not access/adhere/comply, what does the programme do to overcome this?";

- Demonstrate how revised programme outputs will be linked to adjustments in inputs, management/partnerships and enhanced capacity for the new measures.

Summary of the programme theory from Step 2	Theory of inequities postulated at the end of Step 5 (include gender, human rights, social determinants of health)	NEW programme theory

Activities applied throughout the different review steps (theory building and theory testing) have highlighted the multiple interrelationships between the mechanisms and the contextual factors. These will be further explored in the course of the other redesign activities, with the aim of making the programme more equity enhancing, and gender responsive and rights based.

Figure 7.4 Logic model of the theories

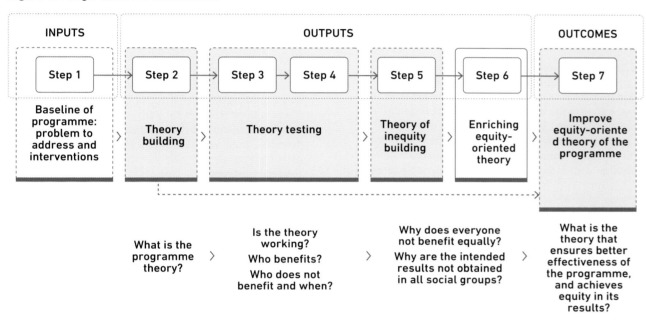

ACTIVITY 2

Identify the scope and level (national, regional, local) of the proposed changes

In this activity the review team describes the specific changes they propose to move from the initial theory described in Step 2 to the new theory (Activity 1 above). These changes to the programme address the mechanisms generating inequities set out in the theory of inequities and achieve more effectiveness in the programme.

This activity includes two tasks:

- Describe the scope and level of the potential programme adjustments; and

- Consider changes that are needed beyond the direct control of the programme and review the expected outcomes of the proposed changes.

STEP 7

2.a. Describe the scope and level of the potential programme adjustments.

In further considering the design and operational reality of the potential changes to the programme, the review team should clarify the scope of the change and the details of the specific adjustments. For more details considering the "scope" of change, please see the related section on this in the background reading for this step.

The "level" of implementation means indicating if the programme adjustments would take place at national, state/province, district and/or local level. Some adjustments that are legislative or regulatory in nature may best be made at national level (e.g. for instance if there is a law that restricts access to certain subpopulations, or the need to regulate actions of another sector like food and agriculture to address

key underlying determinants of health). Some of the influences or policy-making decisions are outside of the programme, but an important contribution of the review team work documented in a report is to give visibility to these aspects. Other adjustments may be more linked to service delivery, at the organization or make changes on activities, and need to respond to specific on-the-ground operational realities, and hence be appropriate for execution, thinking of changes at regional/state or local levels.

Spaces need to be created where stakeholders from different parts of the programme (at national and subnational levels) can discuss the advantages of the proposed changes for both the programme and the subpopulations being considered. To the extent possible, these would be integrated into ongoing existing programme review or implementation-related meetings.

Scope of the proposed adjustment	Potential adjustment (specific change)	Level of implementation (local, regional, national)
Modification of programme contents		
Structural and organizational changes		
Management and financing improvements		
Human resource adjustments		
Normative/standard-setting, regulation or legislation advancements		
Mechanism to involve other sectors with which interventions or activities should be jointly conducted		
Mechanism to empower the priority subpopulation		

2.b. Consider changes that are needed beyond the direct control of the programme.

There will be some barriers and social determinants that the health programme alone will not be able to address, and this will require liaising with other parts of the ministry of health and with other sectors (including through the establishment of official agreements). Suggesting adjustments to a programme will require consultations with stakeholders in the health sector and beyond to explore feasibility, get buy-in and build partnerships. The processes leading to the proposal for redesign must be participatory and open to discussion and debate. In this task, the review team will consider:

• Needed changes that involve and/or have implications for other parts of the health system; and

• Needed changes to the programme that involve engagement of other sectors/cross-government representatives.

Partnering with other parts of the health system: Beyond the direct programme being reviewed, it will likely be important to liaise with stakeholders in other parts of the health system that are implicated by the proposed adjustments (i.e. that may manage human resource training, retention, deployment; financial protection schemes; essential medicines, etc.). In the following box, please describe who these stakeholders are and the implications for their work, and how they can be engaged/consulted in exploring the feasibility of the changes.

Partnering with other sectors and civil society: With regard to engaging other sectors and civil society, quickly review the team's answers to the exercises in Step 6. If other sectors did not participate in the review process from the beginning, it is of great importance to consider inviting them to participate in Steps 7 and 8, as this provides an opportunity for collaboration in the redesign. Further consulting with representatives of the subpopulation communities impacted by the proposed changes is also important. In the following box, please propose an approach to consultation on the suggested intersectoral and social participation components that are part of the emerging redesign proposal (building on your answers to Step 6).

STEP 7

PRODUCE A REDESIGN PROPOSAL TO ACT ON THE REVIEW FINDINGS
STEP 7

ACTIVITY 3

Finalize the revised diagram and theory of the programme to be more equity enhancing and gender responsive and rights based

The review team should then consider how the **programme diagram** initially developed in Step 2 might be adapted for adjustments aimed at addressing the theory of inequities from Step 5, so that it reflects the **new theory of the programme** (a key focus in Step 7). The diagram should be updated with the new or amended interventions and activities, differentiating the original elements from the new elements, for example by using different colours. The revised programme diagram should be congruent with the previous revisions and take into account the specific proposed changes.

It is important to consider each key stage of the programme, thinking about the necessary changes in each of them. Adjustments should be made across the results chain as relevant, including to the inputs, the activities of each key stage, and how these changes modify the outputs. The review team should then define the revised outcomes of the programme, based on the sequences of new/modified activities and mechanisms, to illustrate how issues of equity, gender, human rights and social determinants have been made explicit. Finally, the review team can modify the final impact/expected longer term results to illustrate that the programme aims to reduce inequities/leave no one behind in its efforts to, for instance, decrease morbidity and mortality.

In the process of developing the programme diagram, key considerations about the new programme theory (a preliminary version of which was drafted in Activity 1) may emerge. The review team should update the new programme theory with these considerations.

ACTIVITY 4

Produce a short-term plan for the implementation of the proposed programme adjustments and redesign

With the final new proposed programme theory and diagram in hand, the review team should develop a preliminary plan which captures how and with what resources/organization the programme adjustments will be developed and formally endorsed to become part of the programme. The plan can include reference to integration of the adjustments into the ongoing planning and review cycles of the programme, and address budgeting and resource allocation issues. The plan can also include proposals for piloting the adjustments before scale up, as appropriate.

4.a. In the following box, please describe the implementation strategy. For example, what is the timeframe for alignment with national planning cycles, the partners, core tasks and piloting or other feasibility studies?

4.b. In the case of developing a pilot, please describe the strategy to capture lessons learned, adapt the plan, scale up and extend coverage?

4.c. In advocating for the adoption/endorsement of the redesign proposal, what are the main arguments to give decision-makers (at highest levels responsible for the programme)? Which would be the first three actions the review team would propose to that authority to implement the proposal?

PRODUCE A REDESIGN PROPOSAL TO ACT ON THE REVIEW FINDINGS
STEP 7

ACTIVITY 5

Produce a report with the redesign proposal

This activity essentially consists of completing a report with the redesign proposal, which will be used to further consult with stakeholders and develop the proposed programme changes. This synthesis of review process outputs is useful for seeing through the analysis to actual programmatic changes and implementation.

The redesign proposal should be presented in a report that synthesizes the decisions and thinking of the review team, backed by the outputs of the Innov8 approach and other information gathered through evidence reviews, etc. The report is an overview that permits the team to disseminate its findings and initial proposals for redesign and their justification. It should be simple, short and direct. Please see the example in Box 7.1.

It is important to emphasize that the process of redesign of a programme goes far beyond the production of a report with the redesign proposal, but it is outside the scope of this handbook to accompany the national review team further. The team may also decide to complement this analysis with more in-depth efforts to assess and integrate gender considerations or human rights.[2] Also, because the factors that drive inequities constantly evolve, the review and redesign of programmes is a continuous process. For this reason, it is very important to look at how to build this type of analysis into the ongoing programme planning, review and monitoring and evaluation cycles (see Step 8).

Box 7.1 Example review team report

1. Introduction, rationale and background to the work of the review team.
2. Overview of the situation of inequities and gender and human rights issues for the selected health topic.
3. Brief description of the current aims, objectives and activities of the programme.
4. Summary of the core findings of the review process Steps 1–8 (as per the "outputs" called for at the end of each of the steps).
5. Delineation of the priorities, aims and objectives for redesign.
6. Inclusion of the revised programme theory and the diagram of the programme with the proposed adjustments highlighted.
7. Description of the proposed scope and level of the programme adjustments.
8. Justification of the redesign proposal (citing the evidence base, criteria for prioritization, findings).
9. Preliminary implementation plan for the proposed, covering the timeframe, partners, core tasks, as well as addressing issues of scaling up.
10. Monitoring and evaluation (including also the outputs from Step 8).
11. Annex: Description of national Innov8 review process, and list of the review team members.

---

[2] There are a number of tools available that can help to assess and integrate gender or rights, including WHO gender tools (e.g. gender assessment tool, gender and health programming checklist, gender-responsive logframe, etc.) and tools by WHO and its parters on human rights (e.g. tool to assess policy coherence on human rights and gender equality in health sector strategies, etc.). Innov8 does not aim to duplicate these tools but complements and links to them where appropriate.

STEP 7 OUTPUT

Congratulations, the review team has completed the analysis for Step 7!

The output summary for Step 7 should cover the following components:

- A brief statement of the new programme theory that is more equity enhancing and gender responsive and rights based.

- A revised logic model diagram, showing the sequence of activities of the programme key stages linked to the outputs and outcomes, that is more equity enhancing and gender responsive and rights based.

- A redesign proposal report that includes the following (see Box 7.1 for more details):

  - A synthesis of the outputs and decisions from Steps 1 to 7, including the information and evidence that informed the thinking of the review team;

  - The new programme theory and logic model diagram of the revised programme;

  - Description of the scope and level (national, regional, local) of the proposed changes, including those beyond the direct control of the programme, within and outside the health sector; and

  - A short-term plan for the implementation of the proposed programme adjustments and redesign, including the tasks required, responsible parties, required resources and preliminary timeframe.

REFERENCES

Asthana S, Halliday J (2006). Developing an Evidence base for policies and interventions to address Health inequalities: The Analysis of "Public Health Regimes". The Milbank Quarterly. 2006;84(3):577–603.

Berrie M (2007). Initiating Phase – Feasibility Study Request and Report (#5 in the series Initiating Phase). Queensland University of Technology. Available: http://www.pmhut.com/initiating-phase-feasibility-study-request-and-report (accessed 22 February 2016).

Byng R, Norman I, Redfern S (2005). Using realistic evaluation to evaluate a practice-level intervention to improve primary healthcare for patients with long-term mental illness. Evaluation. 2005;11(1):69–93.

Carrera C, Azrack A, Begkoyian G, Pfaffmann J, Ribaira E, O'Connell T, Doughty P, Aung KM, Prieto L, Rasanathan K, Sharkey A (2012). The comparative cost-effectiveness of an equity-focused approach to child survival, health, and nutrition: a modelling approach. Lancet. 2012;380(9850):1341–1351. Available: http://dx.doi.org/10.1016/S0140-6736(12)61378-6 (accessed 4 March 2016).

Dunn JR, van der Meulen E, O'Campo P and Muntaner C (2013). Improving health equity through theory-informed evaluations: a look at housing first strategies, cross-sectoral health programs, and prostitution policy. Evaluation and Program Planning. 2013;36(1):184–90. Available: http://www.sciencedirect.

com/science/article/pii/S0149718912000250 (accessed 26 February 2016).

Gwatkin DR, Ergo A (2011). Universal health coverage: Friend or foe of health equity? Lancet. 2011;377:2160–2161. doi: 10.1016/S0140-6736(10)62058-2.

Kenny N, Joffres C (2008). An Ethical Analysis of International Health Priority-Setting. Health Care Analysis. 2008;16:145–160.

Lacouture A, Breton E, Guichard A, Ridde V (2015). The concept of mechanism from a realist approach: a scoping review to facilitate its operationalization in public health program evaluation. Implementation Science. 2015;10(1):153. Available: http://www.implementationscience.com/content/10/1/153 (accessed 18 February 2016).

Macintyre S, Chalmers I, Horton R, Smith R (2001). Using evidence to inform health policy: case study. British Medical Journal. 2001;322:222–5.

Marmot M, Allen J, Goldblatt P, et al (2010). Fair Society, Healthy Lives: Strategic Review of Health Inequalities in England post-2010. London: United Kingdom. The Marmot Review.

Ministerio de Salud (2010). Documento Técnico III: Guía para Aanaliza Equidad en el Acceso y los Resultados de los Programas y su Relación con los Determinantes Sociales de la Salud. Serie de Documentos Técnicos del Rediseño de los Programas desde la Perspectiva de Equidad y Determinantes

STEP 7

Sociales. Subsecretaría de Salud Pública: Santiago. [Ministry of Health of Chile (2010). Technical document III for supporting the review and redesign of public health programmes from the perspective of equity and social determinants of health. Santiago: Undersecretary for Public Health.] Materials in Spanish only.

Ministry of Health and Population, Nepal (2016). Review of the national ASRH programme to address equity, social determinants of health, gender and human rights. Final report prepared by Health Research and Social Development Forum (HERD).

Ministry of Health, Social Services and Equality, Government of Spain (2012). Methodological guide to integrate equity into health strategies, programmes and activities. Version 1. Madrid. Available: http://www.msssi.gob.es/profesionales/saludPublica/prevPromocion/promocion/desigualdadSalud/jornadaPresent_Guia2012/docs/Methodological_Guide_Equity_SPAs.pdf (accessed 17 February 2016).

Pawson R, Tilley N (1997). Realistic evaluation. London: Sage.

Pawson R, Tilley N (2004). Realist evaluation. London: British Cabinet Office. Available: http://www.communitymatters.com.au/RE_chapter.pdf (accessed 18 February 2016).

Portillo I, Idigoras I, Bilbao I, Hurtado JL, Urrejola M, Calvo B, Mentxaka A, Hurtado JK (2015). Programa de cribado de cáncer colorectal de euskadi. Centro Coordinador del Programa de Cribado, Subdirección de Asistencia Sanitaria, Dirección General de Osakidetza, Bilbao. Available: http://www.osakidetza.euskadi.eus/contenidos/informacion/deteccion_cancer/es_cancer/adjuntos/programa.pdf (accessed 17 February 2016).

Potts H, Hunt PH (2008). Participation and the right to the highest attainable standard of health. Project Report. Colchester, Essex: Human Rights Centre. Available: http://repository.essex.ac.uk/9714/ (accessed 22 February 2016).

Rychetnik L, Frommer M, Hawe P, Shiell A (2002). Criteria for Evaluating Evidence on Public Health Interventions. Journal of Epidemiology and Community Health. 2002;56:119–27.

UN (2008). Report of the Special Rapporteur on the right of everyone to the enjoyment of the highest attainable standard of physical and mental health. Paul Hunt. New York: Human Rights Council. Available: http://www.who.int/medicines/areas/human_rights/A_HRC_7_11.pdf (accessed 26 February 2016).

WHO (2014). Making fair choices on the path to universal health coverage. Final report of the WHO Consultative Group on Equity and Universal Health Coverage. Geneva: World Health Organization. Available: http://apps.who.int/iris/bitstream/10665/112671/1/9789241507158_eng.pdf?ua=1 (accessed 26 February 2016).

Step8

Strengthen monitoring and evaluation

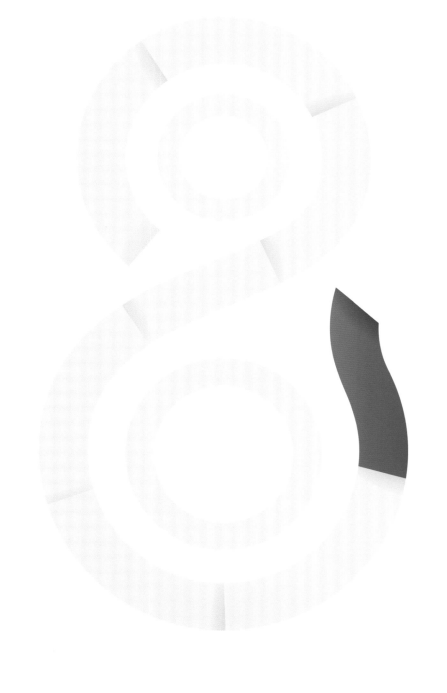

Overview

In Step 8, the review team considers how the Innov8 review and redesign process has resulted in changes (both to the programme and to attitudes and skills of the review team), as well as how the programme's monitoring and evaluation can determine whether the changes are reaching their intended aims. Step 8 also contributes to strengthening the programme's ongoing review, planning, monitoring and evaluation processes. In doing so, Step 8 reinforces a sustained approach to addressing equity, gender, human rights and social determinants of health.

In reaching this step, the review team has carried out what is essentially an evaluative process. Step 8 therefore constitutes a good moment to reflect more broadly on how this process has exerted influence at individual, interpersonal and collective levels. This includes assessing the changes produced in the participants and the programme that contribute to sustained responsiveness to the changing landscape of health inequities.

The central focus of Step 8 for the review team is to consider critical questions including: *How can we monitor if the improved, equity-oriented, gender responsive and rights-based programme is really reaching the intended subpopulation(s) and achieving the expected short-, intermediate and long-term outcomes?* This response involves reflection on indicators, quantitative and qualitative methods and other mechanisms. In doing this, the review team must indicate the timeline of expected results: *When is this new programme likely to show results and have an impact?*

Step 8 includes three activities:

1) Reflecting on how the Innov8 process has exerted influence;

2) Outlining a plan to monitor and evaluate the new programme theory; and,

3) Considering how regular/routine programme planning and review processes can better integrate equity, gender, human rights and social determinants of health.

The main output of Step 8 is the proposal to monitor whether the redesigned programme reaches the priority subpopulations and achieves the intended results, and improves the health programme's monitoring and evaluation framework. This gets integrated into the redesign proposal produced as an output of the redesign proposal (Step 7).

Objectives of Step 8

> Consider how engagement in the Innov8 process has exerted influence and leveraged change for the individual review team members, their interactions and at the collective level of the programme and institution.

> Outline a proposal to monitor whether the revised programme really does reach the priority subpopulations and achieves the intended results.

> Identify inputs from across the review cycle that may be relevant for improving the health programme's monitoring and evaluation framework.

BACKGROUND READING FOR STEP 8

Making evaluation matter: Towards equity-oriented, gender responsive and rights-based monitoring and evaluative processes

The Innov8 approach is based on realist evaluation principles set out in previous sections and draws heavily on Sridharan´s thinking (Sridharan, 2014a), as well as work by WHO on strengthening health information systems to better address equity, gender, human rights and social determinants. It takes from and is consistent with the WHO approach to evaluation, specifically in relation to:

- A focus on expected and achieved accomplishments, examining the results chain, processes, contextual factors and causality, in order to understand achievements or the lack thereof;

- The aim to determine the relevance, impact, effectiveness, efficiency and sustainability of the interventions and institutional contributions;

- Provision of evidence-based information that is credible, reliable and useful, enabling the timely incorporation of findings, recommendations and lessons learned into the decision-making and management processes;

- Forming an integral part of each stage of the strategic planning and programming cycle and not only an end-of-programme activity (WHO 2013); and

- Ensuring that a programme's ongoing monitoring and evaluation (M&E) framework and information system provide the information necessary to monitor who is being missed and benefiting less by the programme on a continual basis, in keeping with commitments to UHC and the SDGs.

Box 8.1 Definitions: monitoring and evaluation

Monitoring: A continuing function that uses systematic collection of data on specified indicators to provide management and the main stakeholders of an ongoing intervention with indications of the extent of progress and achievement of objectives and progress in the use of allocated funds.

Evaluation: The systematic and objective assessment of an ongoing or completed project, programme or policy, its design, implementation and results. The aim is to determine the relevance and fulfilment of objectives, development efficiency, effectiveness, impact and sustainability. An evaluation should provide information that is credible and useful, enabling the incorporation of lessons learned into the decision-making process.

Source: OECD, 2010.

An important aspect of an evaluation process focuses on how people and organizations have become influenced because of the process (Figure 8.1).

For example, as a result of their engagement in the Innov8 approach, it is expected that participants' attitudes about their programme and their understanding of the salience of equity, gender, human rights and social determinants of health issues will develop. It is expected that they will have acquired or strengthened skills to act as agents of change to persuade others. Collectively, at the programme and organizational levels, the process should influence agenda-setting, policy-oriented learning and, ultimately, specific policy and programme changes.

Figure 8.1 How do evaluations exert influence?

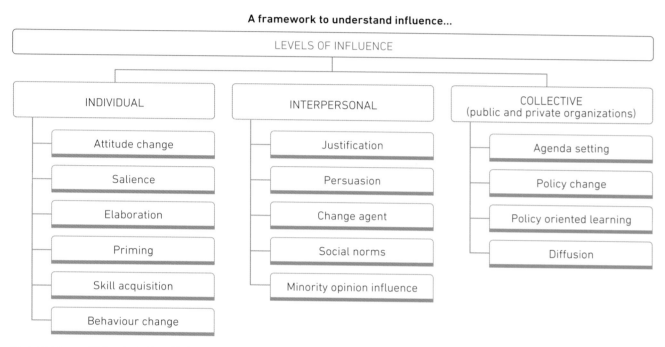

A framework to understand influence...

LEVELS OF INFLUENCE

INDIVIDUAL
- Attitude change
- Salience
- Elaboration
- Priming
- Skill acquisition
- Behaviour change

INTERPERSONAL
- Justification
- Persuasion
- Change agent
- Social norms
- Minority opinion influence

COLLECTIVE
(public and private organizations)
- Agenda setting
- Policy change
- Policy oriented learning
- Diffusion

Source: Sridharan, 2014a, adapted from Mark and Henry, 2004.

Considerations for monitoring and evaluation design of the improved programme

The expected outcome of the Innov8 approach is an improved programme theory that addresses the subpopulations being missed, barriers, mechanisms driving inequities, etc., uncovered in the review process. A critical question is how do we know if this new programme really works? In considering a monitoring and evaluation strategy to answer this question the review team should strike a balance in being rigorous and pragmatic. As Sridharan states, there is no need to seek the "Rolls-Royce" method of causal inference; it is enough to consider a strategic mix of feasible methods that together will give teams enough evidence to say that the new programme is contributing to greater equity – or not (Sridharan, 2016).

Contribution analysis is one approach that allows for real-life, achievable evaluations to help programme managers arrive at conclusions about the contribution their programme has made to the particular outcomes and reduce uncertainty. This approach aligns well with the Innov8 approach in that it considers the observed results through the understanding of why they occurred or did not and the relationships with the intervention and other influences. In other words, it starts from the reasoned theory of the intervention – the programme theory with the key assumptions about why the programme is expected to work, supported by evidence that was developed in the redesign, Step 7. It can be reasonably argued that the intervention has a reasonable contribution causal claim if:

- It was implemented as set out in the programme theory;

- The chain of activities – outputs and outcomes occurred; and

STRENGTHEN MONITORING AND EVALUATION
STEP 8

• Other influencing factors are assessed and their contribution deemed insignificant or recognized (they may be part of the assumptions of the programme theory) (Mayne, 2011).

Specifically, in relation to evaluating interventions that are health equity enhancing, address social determinants, and are rights-based and gender responsive, some relevant questions for reflection are featured below (Sridharan, 2012b; Tannahill & Sridharan, 2013).

How can the monitoring and evaluation design help assess the impacts of an intervention?

Ideally, the design would integrate both monitoring and evaluation approaches. Monitoring aims to study progress against selected indicators and measures the system indicators' headway against targeted goals. Evaluations, on the other hand, study the "why" or "why not" of performance and attempt to provide remedial action if the performance is not up to expectations.

Some elements to consider in designing a monitoring and evaluation plan to determine whether the improved intervention is actually impacting health equities should include:

• Reflection on what successful results (outcomes and longer term impacts) means for an intervention;

• Clarity on the timeline and also a "trajectory" of impact (Woolcock, 2009, cited in Tannahill & Sridharan, 2013);

• Clear and reliable measures – the measures need to be informed by the equity-oriented, gender responsive and rights-based theory;

• Measures of the dynamic contexts that might be necessary for the intervention to work; and

• Discussion on the uses and potential influence of the monitoring and evaluation results.

How can we demonstrate emergent, dynamic learning about the programme as it is implemented?

A standard view of M&E is a linear path. Yet, in monitoring complex interventions, especially when something new and bold is being tried, the path is no longer linear. A more dynamic relationship between the theory, methods and results is involved. To enable a continuous learning process, a range of methods are applied. These may include stratified indicators, exploratory qualitative techniques, and longitudinal follow up.

Figure 8.2 Learning from evaluation methods for continual programme improvement

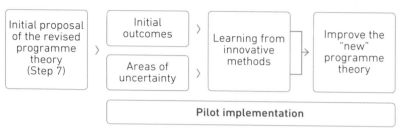

Sources: Sridharan, 2012a; Sridharan 2012b, with modifications by authors.

The "so what?" How did the new initiative improve lives?

One key idea is that good evaluations are eventually about performance stories. The most credible performance stories reflect on how and why investments in interventions make a difference in the lives of individuals, especially those in greatest need. Using qualitative methods to describe perspectives and experiences is one compelling way to tell these performance stories (Sridharan & Nakaima, 2011).

Consider how the review cycle has produced insights for strengthening M&E

Relevant findings from the review cycle, across steps and including the recommended programme adjustments may prove useful to map ways in which the programme M&E framework could be enhanced by integrating equity, gender, human rights and social determinants in ongoing programme planning and review processes.

Figure 8.3 Potential inputs of Innov8 to an M&E framework

Step 3: Identify who is being left out by the programme	› Information on relevant equity stratifiers
Step 4: Consider the barriers and facilitating factors	› Information on barriers that could be monitored
Step 5: Identify mechanisms generating inequities	› Information on core social determinants that could be tracked
Step 6: Consider intersectoral action and social participation	› Process indicators on intersectoral action and participation
Step 7: Produce a redesign proposal for the programme	› Indicators for new interventions and/or targets for equity in coverage of existing interventions

STEP 8

STRENGTHEN MONITORING AND EVALUATION
STEP 8

The checklist of Step 1 asked about the M&E framework for the programme. In a way, those answers are the baseline upon which you can then consider improvements, taking into account critical elements of the programme theory developed in Step 2.

Step 3: Identify who is being left out by the programme

> Information on relevant equity stratifiers

Step 3 on "identifying who is being left out by the programme" asked:

• For the review team's reflections of subpopulations who do not access/benefit at each key stage.

• If existing available quantitative and qualitative data confirm the findings from the review team's reflections.

The answers to these questions can provide orientations for how to improve the M&E framework and, potentially, the data sources behind it. The result would be that key indicators could be disaggregated by the equity stratifiers deemed most appropriate. It is noted that often individual health programmes can have limited decision-making power over data sources such as cross-cutting household surveys, which may provide information reflected in the programme M&E framework. Health programmes nevertheless can advocate for appropriate sample sizes, disaggregation approaches, equity analysis and reporting.

Step 4: Consider the barriers and facilitating factors

> Information on barriers that could be monitored

It may be relevant to also consider adding to the programme M&E framework specific barriers that have emerged in Step 4 of the review process. For instance, if financial barriers, gender-related barriers or discrimination based on ethnicity have emerged as prominent barriers in Step 4, indicators on these can be integrated into the programme M&E framework. This may also entail some adaptation to data sources, or simply the better use of existing data.

Step 5: Identify mechanisms generating inequities

> Information on core social determinants that could be tracked

---

In Step 5, the review team may have identified key underlying determinants relevant to the programme and the health topic it addresses. For instance, if poverty and education levels were identified as being critical to explaining health inequities, these could be tracked by the programme for the target population. The programme would not necessarily have to collect data on these, but rather could track them through different sources (for example from surveys conducted by other sectors).

Step 6: Consider intersectoral action and social participation

> Process indicators on intersectoral action and participation

---

The review team, through Step 6, may have identified that there were key programme inputs and process issues, such as joint actions conducted with another sector or consultations held with the target population, among other participation mechanisms, that are necessary for improving how the programme tackles health inequities. The review team can consider if process/input indicators reflecting these have a place in the programme's M&E framework.

> Indicators for new interventions and/or targets for equity in coverage of existing interventions

Finally, in the redesign Step 7, the review team will have delineated changes to the programme to enable it to reduce inequities. These changes, which can constitute new activities or interventions or the amendment of existing ones, can be reflected in the M&E framework. Also, if the redesign has resulted in identification of equity targets to help close coverage gaps for disadvantaged subpopulations, this is the chance to integrate those into the programme M&E framework.

Beyond just looking at the indicators of the M&E framework, the review team can also look at the M&E processes. It is important to orchestrate programme-related monitoring in a way that is participatory, transparent and ensures confidentiality, in keeping with a HRBA (UN, 2012). This applies to both qualitative and quantitative data sources, as well as how data is stored/protected, analysed, reported and used. For instance, this may mean involving representatives from the target population in the analysis and reporting of data, ensuring the adequate personal identity protection measures (e.g. for data disaggregated by race/ethnicity), and featuring data and reports in the public domain.

Building the capacity of programme staff in analysis, reporting, and dissemination and use of information on health inequalities may be a necessary step. Proficiency in analysing health inequality data requires not only technical knowledge of the measures and calculations, but also an awareness of the best practices of how analyses are applied and interpreted (WHO, 2013; WHO, 2014; WHO, 2015). WHO is now working on demonstrating best practices in reporting the results of health inequality monitoring, to introduce innovative, interactive ways for audiences to explore inequality data. It also has available capacity-building resources and normative guidance that can be of support to the programme staff (see http://www.who.int/gho/health_equity/videos/en/).

Many of the changes to the programme M&E framework and processes will take consultation with experts, sometimes in data and statistics divisions of the government, who may not be included in the review team. Finalizing a proposal for changes to the M&E framework can entail consultation with them.

Consider how regular/routine programme reviews might better integrate equity, gender, human rights and social determinants of health

The regular/ongoing planning and review processes for a health programme will depend very much on the country and programme context. Reviews (and related planning activities) may be informed from the ground up, with district reviews, province/state reviews and a national review of progress.

Understanding a programme planning and review cycle requires mapping:

• The assessment approach and components of the planning and review process, including in relation to the programme's M&E framework;

• How the review is conducted at the different levels – district, subnational and national – and the information flows between them;

• The sequencing of the review components and the timeline for planning;

• The information sources and instruments for information collection (quantitative and qualitative, state and non-state);

• The oversight body for the review, the coordination mechanisms, and the stakeholders consulted (beyond the programme staff), including the extent to which men and women from diverse groups participated equally;

- How findings are analysed, prioritized and reported;

- How findings are used in planning and budgeting;

- How final decisions are made in the planning process and the criteria for these; and

- How findings of programme-specific reviews/planning feed into wider health sector reviews and planning processes (e.g. for national health plans).

The review team can consider entry points for adjustments to the ongoing planning and review processes of the programme to ensure that there are embedded mechanisms to continuously address health inequities, gender and human rights. Example adjustments include:

- Use of equity-relevant information in reviews and planning (see previous section on the M&E framework);

- Involvement of women and men from disadvantaged subpopulations in consultations to inform review and planning exercises;

- Consultation with other sectors in review and planning processes; and

- Incorporation of relevant criteria in exercises related to prioritization of activities and budgeting, to leave no one behind (and ensure that the programme performs at least as well for the most disadvantaged subpopulations as it does for the more advantaged subpopulations).

Step 8 Additional reading and resources

WHO (2011). Monitoring, evaluation and review of national health strategies. A country-led platform for information and accountability. Geneva: World Health Organization. Available: http://www.who.int/healthinfo/country_monitoring_evaluation/1085_IER_131011_web.pdf (accessed 24 February 2016).

WHO (2013). Handbook on health inequality monitoring – with a special focus on low- and middle-income countries. Geneva: World Health Organization. Available: http://apps.who.int/iris/bitstream/10665/85345/1/9789241548632_eng.pdf (accessed 24 February 2016).

WHO (2014). Monitoring health inequality: An essential step for achieving health equity. Geneva: World Health Organization. Available: http://apps.who.int/iris/bitstream/10665/133849/1/WHO_FWC_GER_2014.1_eng.pdf (accessed 26 February 2016).

Videos: Monitoring health inequality: illustrations of fundamental concepts http://www.who.int/gho/health_equity/videos/en/

CASE STUDY EXAMPLES OF STEP 8 EVALUATION LEARNINGS AND MONITORING AND EVALUATION OF REDESIGN PROPOSALS

Nepal's M&E framework for the redesign proposal of the national adolescent sexual and reproductive health programme

After developing its programme review process, Nepal's national ASRH programme reflected on some of the influences at individual and collective level. First of all, the process enabled participants to identify the hidden barriers to obtaining the programme results found in the theory of inequities.

As a result, the new programme theory was considered to be more focused on equity and enriched with interventions expected to improve the quality of the ASRH programme and its implementation in the Nepalese context, which should lead to further availability, accessibility and coverage of services for all adolescents, especially those from the most vulnerable groups, such as adolescents living in rural areas and urban slums.

The importance of collaboration with different stakeholders and of social participation was recognized by all participants in the review process and, institutionally, will be adopted as an integral practice in the future during development and implementation of the ASRH programme as well as the broader adolescent health and development strategy. In addition, the process offered an opportunity to create strong networks and alliances between participants.

For the participants, the most important benefit was the realization that the success of every intervention could be compromised if the issues of context and heterogeneity that result in vulnerable groups facing specific needs and confronting specific barriers are not taken into consideration. Thus, identifying and overcoming these aspects was integral to the development and implementation of pro-equity interventions.

In addition to considering the influences of the Innov8 approach, the Nepal team considered how to monitor whether the main adjustments to the revised programme really would reach the prioritized subpopulation – youth living in rural areas – and achieve the expected results (see Table 8.1).

Table 8.1 Nepal´s national ASRH programme M&E framework for the main adjustments

Input/process indicators	Activities	Output indicators	Outcome indicators	Impact
Adolescent friendly services (AFS) site selection criteria revised Number of AFS established	Planning intersectoral coordination for selection of AFS sites	Number of AFSs established in rural hard-to-reach areas	Number of adolescents receiving services from AFSs disaggregated by age, sex, ethnicity, education, urban/rural, wealth quintile etc.	Age at marriage increased Contraceptive prevalence rate increased Unmet need decreased Adolescent pregnancy decreased Age-specific fertility rate among adolescents decreased Reproductive health related morbidities and mortality decreased among adolescents
Number of training sessions for service providers	Trainings for service providers	Number of trained service providers disaggregated by sex and geography	Number of AFS providing quality AFS Number/% of adolescents who perceive that providers deliver service with discrimination	Number/% of adolescents who are aware of and use AFS disaggregated by age, sex, ethnicity, education, urban/rural, wealth quintile etc.
Number of schools containing adolescent information corners	Implementation of corners with adequate education and behaviour (IEC/behavioural change communication – BCC) materials at adolescent information corner	Number of adolescent information corner containing adequate IEC/BCC materials	Number of adolescents / teachers using IEC/BCC materials from adolescent information corner	
Revision of guidelines prepared by Management Division ensuring the mandatory participation of adolescents in health facility operation and management committee (HFOMC)	Participation of adolescents in HFOMC and ASRH related programme	Number of HFOMC including adolescent members, disaggregated by sex and age	Number of HFOMC including adolescent members, disaggregated by sex and age	Number/% of adolescents who are empowered to practise their rights, disaggregated by age, sex, ethnicity, education, urban/rural, wealth quintile etc.

Source: Ministry of Health and Population of Nepal,2016.

Evaluation of lessons learned from the programme review process in Chile

In 2009–2010, the programme review methodology used in Chile was developed and owned by six different health programme managers working in review teams, called "nodes", to evoke networks for change. The review teams, led by the managers, included local level programme managers and frontline providers, managers from other related health programmes, intersectoral actors and civil society representatives. The review and redesign process was inspired by the concepts of critical and realistic assessment, particularly Sridharan's guidelines related to theory-based evaluation, considering the concepts that a good evaluator must apply.

What was unique about the Chilean programme review process (2009–2010)?

It developed a dynamic process, involving multiple public health programmes to collectively reflect on how to address unmet population needs and health inequities through programme adjustments, intersectoral action and participation, using a health equity and social determinants of health perspective, characterized by:

- A process developed and owned by key stakeholders (six programme review teams working as nodes in a network for change);

- Focus on action/solutions; with measurable results in terms of programme changes and outcomes;

- Strong political and policy backing;

- Remarkable progress in one year; and

- Served as an example for many other processes in many countries.

Nevertheless, five years later with a new review process beginning in Chile, the Ministry of Health considered how to further embed evaluative thinking

Source: Sridharan, 2014b.

into both the process and ongoing programme planning and evaluation cycles. The following questions were discussed as important in documenting and analysing:

- What are the lessons learned about: (i) changes to perceptions of the problem(s) of the programme and the types of solutions required to overcome them; (ii) the benefits and challenges of intersectoral action; and (iii) social participation; and importantly, (iv) understanding the gaps in the process?

- What are the chains of influence of the initiative and how did they work at individual and collective levels? Have they persisted and deepened?

- What about spheres of control? How much leverage does a redesign proposal alone have (before endorsement, piloting and all of the other necessary work to see things through to actual changes on the ground)?

- What structures/types of support were provided and are needed for the review and redesign process?

- What changes in programme results can be linked to the redesign?

- What are the objects to monitor and evaluate: recommendations/actions/lessons learned/ outcomes?

- What is the impact timeline? When will the changes in outcomes be expected?

- Was a common language and purpose established across sectors to facilitate changes and indicators needed to overcome boundaries with partners?

- Did the revised programme really succeed in reaching those most in need?

- What innovations in planning, adjustments in ongoing M&E frameworks and strategic learning occurred and can be shared?

STEP 8 ACTIVITIES SUMMARY

The activities of Step 8 are summarized in Table 8.2.

Table 8.2 **Summary of activities to develop Step 8: Strengthen monitoring and evaluation**

Questions	Tasks	Methods
Activity 1: Reflect on how the Innov8 process has exerted influence		
What attitudes, skills and changes have resulted in the review team and other levels from the process?	• Discussion of the levels of influence the process has exerted on review team members as individuals, their interpersonal relations and collectively at the programme or institutional level.	Team discussion
Activity 2: Outline a plan to monitor and evaluate the revised programme theory		
How do we know if the revised programme is reaching and benefiting women and men from the intended subpopulation(s)?	• Discuss the considerations from the reading and identify feasible ways to measure the programme outputs and outcomes with a focus on leaving no one behind.	Team discussion Consideration of planning and programme cycle requirements: information and timeline
Activity 3: Consider how regular/routine programme planning and review processes can better integrate equity, gender, human rights and social determinants of health		
What insights for enhancing the programme's monitoring and evaluation framework have emerged during the process?	• Review the considerations in the reading and identify relevant aspects to be considered.	Team discussion

STEP 8 ACTIVITY GUIDE

This section outlines the activities to complete after the training in order to finalize your outputs for this element of the redesign phase.

ACTIVITY 1

Reflect on how the Innov8 process has exerted influence

1. **Considering Figure 8.1, the review team should consider what changes have occurred as result of participating in the review and redesign process**.

Individual level	Interpersonal level	Collective (for the programme and the institution)

STRENGTHEN MONITORING AND EVALUATION
STEP 8

ACTIVITY 2

Outline a plan to monitor and evaluate the revised programme theory (outcome of Step 7)

In this activity, the review team will look at the revised programme theory of the improved, equity-oriented, gender and rights responsive programme and discuss the following questions. The answers should be briefly summarized.

2.a. How will we know if the changes introduced in the programme will produce the expected results?

2.b. What key inputs, outputs and outcomes of the review programme need to be monitored? How? When should they be measured (new interventions or activities)?

Key input, output or outcome	How can it be monitored?	When?

If the answer to how considers indicators, will these be quantitative and qualitative? Identify the relevant stratifiers.

In terms of when, often it is important to obtain information quickly to share with high-level directors, stakeholders and to re-orient interventions, even if it is only indicative and not definitive.

Capacity-building

2.c. With regard to analysis, reporting, dissemination and use of data on health inequalities (and on barriers and determinants), what kind of capacity exists?

- Are there resources available for analysis, reporting and dissemination?

- Do staff have the necessary knowledge and skills, including on equity, gender, human rights and social determinants of health?

- If not, what changes may be needed and what inputs are needed to activate them?

ACTIVITY 3

Consider how regular/routine programme planning and review processes can better integrate equity, gender, human rights and social determinants of health

3.a. Please refer back to the review team's findings on the checklist (see Step 1), in particular the questions on monitoring. With these in hand, consider the following table and questions, which aim to assist the review team to see how the findings from the review cycle may be relevant to enhance monitoring from an equity, gender, human rights and social determinants perspective.

Remember, the idea is not to mechanically fill in all of these boxes but to identify aspects that might be relevant to strengthen the programme's monitoring and evaluation framework. Keep in mind the acronym for surveillance systems: KISS (keep it simple and sensitive).

Component of the review cycle	Question on relevance for the programme's M&E framework	What emerges as relevant from your findings
Step 3: Identify who is being left out by the programme	Are there equity stratifiers that should be included? If stratification is not possible, what other data sources could capture information for specific subpopulations?	
Step 4: Consider the barriers and facilitating factors that subpopulations experience	If not done so already, is there a need to systematically monitor any of the key barriers identified?	
Step 5: Identify the mechanisms that generating inequities	Which social determinants of health should be tracked? Structural and/or intermediary social determinants?	
Step 6: Explore how intersectoral action and social participation can be used to reduce inequities	Are there relevant indicators for social participation and intersectoral action that should be added?	

STEP 8 OUTPUTS

Congratulations, the review team has completed the analysis for Step 8!

The review team should **summarize the outputs of Step 8 in a short report (approximately two to five pages)**, while this analysis is fresh in your minds. The output summary should clearly and succinctly capture the main findings and decisions of the review team across the activities in this step. You should integrate the findings from this step into the "redesign proposal report" (see Step 7 example – Box 7.1).

The output summary for Step 8 should cover the following components:

- A description of how the Innov8 process has exerted influence over the review team.

- An outline of a plan to monitor and evaluate the revised programme theory.

- A summary of considerations on how regular/routine programme planning and review processes can better integrate equity, gender, human rights and social determinants.

REFERENCES

Mark M and Henry G (2004). The mechanisms and outcomes of evaluation influence. Evaluation. 2004; 10(1): 35-57. Available: http://evi.sagepub.com/content/10/1/35.abstract (accessed 10 August 2016).

Mayne J (2011). Contribution analysis: Addressing cause and effect. In: Forss K, Marra M, Schwartz R, eds. Evaluating the complex: Attribution, contribution and beyond. 18:53–96. New Brunswick, New Jersey: Transaction Publishers.

Ministry of Health and Population, Nepal (2016). Review of the national ASRH programme to address equity, social determinants of health, gender and human rights. Final report prepared by Health Research and Social Development Forum (HERD).

OECD (2010). Glossary of key terms in evaluation and results based management. Available: http://www.oecd.org/development/evaluation/2754804.pdf (accessed 27 February 2016).

Ottersen OP, Dasgupta J, Blouin C, Buss P, Chongsuvivatwong V, Frenk J, Fukuda-Parr S, Gawanas BP, Giacaman R, Gyapong J, Leaning J (2014). The political origins of health inequity: prospects for change. Lancet. 2014;383(9917):630–667. Available: http://www.thelancet.com/journals/lancet/article/PIIS0140-6736(13)62407-1/fulltext (accessed 27 February 2016).

Sridharan S (2012a). Understanding and Evaluating Complex Programs and Policies. Presentation Ontario CES Meeting. Ontario, Canada. Available: http://evaluationontario.ca/wp-content/uploads/2012/11/Sanjeev-Sridharan-Understanding-and-Evaluating-Complex-Programs.pdf (accessed 24 February 2016).

Sridharan S (2012b). A Pocket Guide to Evaluating Health Equity Interventions – Some Questions for Reflection by Sanjeev Sridharan. Magic: Measuring & Managing Access Gaps in Care (blog entry). Available: http://www.longwoods.com/blog/a-pocket-guide-to-evaluating-health-equity-interventions-some-questions-for-reflection/ (accessed 17 February 2016).

Sridharan S (2014a). Making Evaluations Matter. Presentation. Santiago, Chile. 2014.

Sridharan S (2014b). Evaluating the redesign process (looking forward): Reflections from a distance. Presentation. Programme review from an equity and SDH perspective workshop. Santiago, Chile: Ministry of Health. April 2014.

Sridharan S (2016). Towards a structured process to evaluate health inequities in complex interventions. Presentation for the Ministry of Health. Santiago, Chile. January 2016.

Sridharan S, Nakaima A (2011). Ten steps to making evaluation matter. Evaluation and Program Planning. 2011;34(2):135–46. doi:10.1016/j.evalprogplan.2010.09.003.

Tannahill C, Sridharan S (2013). Getting real about policy and practice needs: evaluation as a bridge between the problem and solution space. Evaluation and Program Planning. 2013;36:157–64. Available: http://www.sciencedirect.com/science/article/pii/S0149718912000213 (accessed: 8 March 2016).

UN (2012). Human Rights Indicators: A guide to measurement and implementation. New York and Geneva: UN Office of the High Commissioner for Human Rights. Available: http://www.ohchr.org/EN/Issues/Indicators/Pages/HRIndicatorsIndex.aspx (accessed 27 February 2016).

WHO (2011). Monitoring, evaluation and review of national health strategies. A country-led platform for information and accountability. Geneva: World Health Organization. Available: http://www.who.int/healthinfo/country_monitoring_evaluation/1085_IER_131011_web.pdf (accessed 24 February 2016).

WHO (2013). Handbook on health inequality monitoring – with a special focus on low- and middle-income countries. Geneva: World Health Organization. Available: http://apps.who.int/iris/bitstream/10665/85345/1/9789241548632_eng.pdf (accessed 24 February 2016).

WHO (2014). Monitoring health inequality: An essential step for achieving health equity. Geneva: World Health Organization. Available: http://apps.who.int/iris/bitstream/10665/133849/1/WHO_FWC_GER_2014.1_eng.pdf (accessed 26 February 2016).

WHO (2015). State of Inequality: reproductive, maternal, newborn and child health. Geneva: World Health Organization. Available: http://apps.who.int/iris/bitstream/10665/164590/1/9789241564908_eng.pdf?ua=1&ua=1 (accessed 24 February 2016).

Woolcock M (2009). Toward a plurality of methods in project evaluation: a contextualised approach to understanding impact trajectories and efficacy. Journal of development effectiveness. 2009;1(1):1–14. Doi: 10.1080/19439340902727719.

Glossary

Glossary of key terms

This glossary provides definitions and brief descriptions of the key concepts, principles and other terms used in the Innov8 approach for reviewing national health programmes and its associated materials and resources, including this Technical Handbook.

Cross references of terms in the glossary are indicated by **bold blue text**.

AAAQ

Acronym for the four interrelated and essential elements of the right to health under Article 12 of the International Covenent on including **Availability**, **Accessibility**, **Acceptability** and **Quality** as outlined in Committee on Economic, Social and Cultural Rights General Comment 14. See the individual terms for their definitions and brief descriptions.

ABC of the programme

The "ABC" of the programme (Pawson & Sridharan, 2009) includes:

a. **Conceptualization and contextualization of the problem to be addressed:** Contextualization of the problem (whether it is a social, institutional or environmental problem) refers to where the health problem occurs and the causal model of the health problem.

b. **What to do**: The changes that must occur to address, reduce or eliminate these problems.

c. **How to do it**: The ideas or actions that are required to bring about new solutions and resources to individuals or communities facing the health problem, so as to bring about the changes that the programme aims at and on which it is based.

Acceptability

Even if resources are available and accessible, they may not be used if the population does not accept them. Acceptability is one of the four elements of the right to health and is means that all health facilities, goods and services must be respectful of medical ethics and culturally appropriate, i.e. respectful of the culture of individuals, minorities, peoples and communities, sensitive to gender and life-cycle requirements, as well as being designed to respect confidentiality and improve the health status of those concerned (CESCR, 2000).

According to Tanahashi, acceptability coverage is influenced by people's perceptions, expectations for health services and personal beliefs. Often, it is based on previous experiences and interactions with health personnel. Discriminative attitudes of health personnel, soliciting of informal payments (or inappropriate use of public services for private gain) by health personnel, and perceptions of low quality services (including safety concerns) can create systemic barriers to acceptability coverage (Tanahashi, 1978).

Accessibility

Even if the service is available, it must be located within reasonable reach of the people who should benefit from it. The capacity of the service is limited by the number of people who can reach and use it and thereby access it (Tanahashi, 1978). There are two main dimensions of accessibility: physical access and financial accessibility.

- **Physical accessibility:** Distance from a health service provider is a strong accessibility factor. Another factor closely related to distance and transport is time. Travel time may be more relevant than distance, as lack of all-weather roads can lead to difficulties in access during monsoon and rains. Mountainous terrain can also prolong travel times, hence creating an access barrier. The travel time to a health facility to access services and the waiting time to see a health professional are associated with the patients' perception of accessibility of services. However, the value of time (the opportunity cost of time) is different for different groups of people and consequently its impact as an access barrier will also vary.

- **Financial accessibility:** User fees and transport costs have been shown to negatively impact access to health services, rendering health services less accessible to poor and vulnerable households. Uncertainty of costs and expectations of high out-of-pocket costs (formal or informal) can also obstruct access. See **Effective coverage** for issues related to financial protection.

As one of the element of the right to health, accessibility means that all health facilities, goods and services have to be accessible to everyone without discrimination, with four broad and overlapping dimensions (see CESCR, 2000):

- **Non-discrimination:** health facilities, goods and services must be accessible to all, especially the most vulnerable or marginalized sections of the population, in law and in fact, without discrimination on any of the prohibited grounds.

- **Physical accessibility:** health facilities, goods and services must be within safe physical reach for all sections of the population.

- **Information accessibility:** the right to seek, receive and impart information and ideas concerning health issues without limiting the right to confidentiality.

- **Economic (of financial) accessibility:** health facilities, goods and services must be affordable for all, including payment for ehalth services as well as the underlying determinants of health.

Accountability

Rights and obligations demand accountability, a key principle of a human rights-based approach. Under international human rights law, duty-bearers are obligated to respect, protect and fulfil human rights, including the right to health and other health-related rights. Accountability compels a State to explain what it is doing and why and how it is moving, as expeditiously and effectively as possible, towards the realization of the right to health for all. Mechanisms of accountability are crucial for ensuring that the State obligations arising from the right to health are respected and that redress options exist to investigate and address alleged violations. The right to health can be realized and monitored through various accountability mechanisms, but as a minimum, all such mechanisms must be accessible, transparent and effective (UN CESCR, 2000; UN CESCR, 2003; WHO, 2013a; WHO, 2014a).

Assessment

Assessment is the process of determining the value or meaning of an activity, policy or programme. Assessment should be systematic and as objective as possible and assess the project, programme or planned policy in terms of its design, implementation and outcomes. The aim of assessment is to determine the relevance and achievement of objectives, efficiency, effectiveness, impact and sustainability of development.

Availability

The ratio between availability of resources – such as human power, facilities, drugs – and the size of the target population gives the measurement of availability coverage (Tanahashi, 1978). Availability coverage considers the resources available for delivering an intervention and their sufficiency, namely the number or density of health facilities and personnel or the availability of necessary inputs (e.g. drugs, equipment). Availability coverage measures the capacity of a health system in relation to the size of the target population or ideally for the population in need.

Availability is one of the elements of the right to health and means functioning public health and health-care facilities, goods and services, as well as programmes, have to be available in sufficient quantity. The precise nature of the facilities, goods and services will vary depending on numerous factors, including the State party's level of development. They will include, however, the underlying determinants of health, such as safe drinking-water and adequate sanitation facilities; hospitals, clinics and other health-related buildings; trained medical and professional personnel receiving domestically competitive salaries; and essential drugs. The availability of services can be affected by how decision-makers choose to allocate resources, based on political priorities or vested interests.

Barriers

In the Tanahashi (1978) effective coverage model, barriers are understood as those factors that hinder the target population from appropriate use of an offered health service or a social guarantee, thus diminishing effective coverage of a health or provision service. Similarly, the right to health draws attention to four types of barriers in access, including physical, financial, information and discrimination barriers. It is important to note that there might be gender-based barriers in access to and use of health services.

Contact coverage

Contact coverage is the actual contact between the service provider and the user. The number of people who have contacted the service is a measure of service output (Tanahashi, 1978). It is similar to "use of services".

Context

Contexts are contingent conditions that may alter the relationship between the programme and outcomes. The context may refer to national policies, community norms, institutional structures and cultural systems. The question is therefore how the programme has taken into consideration these context issues in its organization and design, and whether the programme has identified actions or interventions to address them. Part of the context is the co-existence of other strategies, policies and programmes, as well as the overarching functionality of levels of the health system. These can influence the programme in synergistic or detrimental ways.

Discrimination

Discrimination is unjust or prejudicial treatment of different categories of people. According to the UN Committee on Economic, Social and Cultural Rights (UN CESCR, 2009), the prohibited grounds of discrimination are identified as "race, colour, sex, language, religion, political or other opinion, national or social origin, property, birth or other status". Discrimination can be in laws, policies and practices (de jure) – e.g. in the distribution and provision of resources and health services; or indirect (de facto) – e.g. policies and actions can lead to inequalities in access and in the enjoyment of rights (WHO & OHCHR, 2015). The prohibition of discrimination does not mean that differences should not be acknowledged. In fact, marginalized groups may require targeted attention to help them catch up with the rest of the population.

Downstream, midstream, upstream interventions

Downstream: Interventions addressing the consequences that the health problem creates,

mainly comprising those interventions related to the secondary prevention, curative, rehabilitative and palliative components of the continuum of care.

Midstream: Interventions aimed at reducing the magnitude of exposures and/or giving greater support to those experiencing more vulnerability to exposure, with these including:

• Interventions for changing behaviours and lifestyles; and
• Interventions on living and working conditions.

Upstream: Interventions that intend to modify the context and/or social stratification, i.e. the distribution of power that leads some social subpopulations to experience a greater degree of exposure and vulnerability (adapted from Ministry of Health, Social Services and Equality, Government of Spain, 2012).

Effective coverage

The Tanahashi model defines effective coverage as the proportion of the population in need of an intervention which received an effective intervention (Tanahashi, 1978). For health interventions that require a one-time action, contact coverage may be virtually equivalent to effective coverage. For other interventions, such as chronic disease treatment, effectiveness can require diagnostic accuracy, provider compliance for evidence-based treatment, "continuity" of access by the patient, effectiveness of referrals, and adherence to prescribed treatment and rehabilitation (WHO, 2010). As this study focuses on **Universal health coverage** (see definition), effective coverage also entails financial protection. Out-of-pocket health expenditure as a percentage of total health expenditure and the percentage of the population suffering from catastrophic health expenditures can be used as indicators to measure financial protection.

Empowerment

Empowerment is a multidimensional social process that enables people to expand their assets and capabilities to participate in, negotiate with, influence, control and hold accountable, institutions that affect their lives (Narayan, 2005). Empowering rights-holders to claim their rights is a precondition for active, free and meaningful participation – one of the principles of a human rights-based approach. Strategies for empowerment therefore often challenge

GLOSSARY OF KEY TERMS

existing power allocations and relations to give disadvantaged groups more power. With respect to women's health, empowerment has often meant, for example, increasing education opportunities and access to relevant information to enable women to make informed decisions about their health, improve self-esteem and equip them with communication and negotiation skills. Such skills are known to influence, for example, safer sex practices, treatment adherence and timely health-seeking behaviour.

Equality and non-discrimination

All individuals are equal as human beings and by virtue of the inherent dignity of each person. All human beings are entitled to their human rights without discrimination of any kind, such as race, colour, sex, ethnicity, age, language, religion, political or other opinion, national or social origin, disability, property, birth or other status as explained by the human rights treaty bodies (UN HRBA Portal, 2016). This necessitates that health services, goods and facilities must be provided to all without discrimination – which is a key dimension of the right to health element of acccessibility.

Equity objective

Equity objectives should specifically seek the reduction or elimination of health differences among social groups or territories (subpopulations) that are systematic and avoidable. Objectives on equity include objectives relevant to action on social determinants of health (including gender) and application of a human rights-based approach in ways that enhance health equity.

Evaluation

Evaluation is the systematic and objective assessment of an ongoing or completed project, programme or policy, its design, implementation and results. The aim is to determine the relevance and fulfilment of objectives, development efficiency, effectiveness, impact and sustainability. An evaluation should provide information that is credible and useful, enabling the incorporation of lessons learned into the decision-making process of both recipients and donors. It is an integral part of each stage of the strategic planning and programming cycle and not only an end-of-programme activity (WHO, 2013b; UNEG, 2012).

Facilitating factors

Those factors helping the target population to benefit from the results expected from the programme, including those that allow for the overcoming of access barriers and achieving an effective use (Ministerio de Salud, Chile, 2010).

Gender

Refers to the socially constructed norms, roles and relationships of and between groups of women, men, boys and girls. Gender also refers to expressions and identities of women, men, boys, girls and gender-diverse people. Gender is inextricable from the social and structural determinants shaping health and equity and can vary across time and place. The concept of gender includes five important elements: relational, hierarchical, historical, contextual and institutional. While most people are born either male or female, they are taught appropriate norms and behaviours – including how they should interact with others of the same or opposite sex within households, communities and workplaces. When individuals or groups do not "fit" established **gender norms, roles or relations**, they often face stigma, discriminatory practices or social exclusion – all of which adversely affect health (WHO, 2011).

Gender mainstreaming

Gender mainstreaming is the process of assessing the implications for women and men of any planned action, including legislation, policies or programmes, in all areas and at all levels. It is a strategy for making women's as well as men's concerns and experiences an integral dimension of the design, implementation, monitoring and evaluation of policies and programmes in all political, economic and societal spheres so that women and men benefit equally and inequality is not perpetuated (WHO, 2011).

Gender norms

Gender norms refer to beliefs about women and men, boys and girls that are passed from generation to generation through the process of socialization. They change over time and differ in different cultures, contexts and populations. Gender norms lead to inequality if they reinforce:

• Mistreatment of one group or sex over the other; or
• Differences in power and opportunities (WHO, 2011).

Gender relations

Gender relations refer to social relations between and among women and men, boys and girls that are based on gender norms and roles. Gender relations often create hierarchies between and among groups of men and women that can lead to unequal power relations, disadvantaging some groups over others (WHO, 2011). At a broader level, gender relations also refer to sociopolitical and economic relations to institutions such as the State, corporations and social movements. This includes the collective processes by which power is mobilized and exercised. Gender relations must be understood in relation to systems and processes such as racism, sexism, homophobia (e.g. discriminatory policies), which shape gender and gendered experiences.

Gender roles

Gender roles refer to what women and men are expected to do (i.e., in the household, community and workplace) in a given society (WHO, 2011).

Health in All Policies (HiAP)

Health in All Policies is an approach to public policies across sectors that systematically takes into account the health implications of decisions, seeks synergies, and avoids harmful health impacts in order to improve population health and health equity (WHO & Ministry of Social Affairs and Health, Government of Finland, 2013; WHO (WHA67.12), 2014b).

Health equity

Equity is the absence of avoidable, unfair or remediable differences among groups of people, whether those groups are defined socially, economically, demographically or geographically or by other means of stratification. "Health equity" or "equity in health" implies that ideally everyone should have a fair opportunity to attain their full health potential and that no one should be disadvantaged from achieving this potential (WHO, 2015a).

Health programme

The joint actions organized around goals and targets for improving the health of the population, usually defined by the ministry of health to make operative a policy to be executed by regional health authorities and/or the health-care networks, and sometimes by other sectors or actors. Consideration of a health programme includes its formulation, implementation process, access to services and outcomes (adapted from Ministry of Health, Social Services and Equality, Government of Spain, 2012).

Health system

A health system is the ensemble of all public and private organizations, institutions and resources mandated to improve, maintain or restore health. Health systems encompass both personal and population services, as well as activities to influence the policies and actions of other sectors to address the social, environmental and economic determinants of health (WHO Regional Office for Europe, 2008).

Heterogeneity of population

Within a population, different subpopulations (as classified by place of residence, sex, socioeconomic status, etc.) have different needs and experiences in terms of exposure to risk factors, health problems and health service access. Compared with the population as a whole, some subpopulations experience greater vulnerability or exposure to health risks and poorer access and outcomes in relation to health services. The health programme must recognize and account for this heterogeneity in terms of the type, formulation and delivery of interventions and activities, as not doing so may directly or indirectly reinforce inequities.

Human rights

Human rights are rights inherent to all human beings and cannot be taken away (they are inalienable). All human beings are equally entitled to their human rights without discrimination, regardless of their nationality, income, place of residence, sex, national or ethnic origin, colour, religion, language, health or other status. Human rights are interrelated, interdependent and indivisible. Universal human rights are often expressed and guaranteed by law, in the forms of international and regional treaties and customary law, regional instruments as well as national constitutions and legislation. International human rights law lays down obligations on governments to act in certain ways or to refrain from certain acts, in order to respect, protect and fulfil human rights and fundamental freedoms of individuals or groups. Also see **Right to health** (OHCHR, 2014).

GLOSSARY OF KEY TERMS

Human rights-based approach

A human rights-based approach (HRBA) to health focuses attention and provides strategies and solutions to redress inequalities, discriminatory practices (both real and perceived) and unjust power relations, which are often at the heart of inequitable health outcomes. The UN Statement of Common Understanding on Human Rights-Based Approaches to Development Cooperation and Programming (2003) aims to ensure that human rights principles inform all programming across all stages of the project cycle, including assessment and analysis, programme planning and design, implementation, monitoring and evaluation (UNDG, 2003). The goal of the HRBA to health is that all health policies, strategies and programmes be designed with the objective of *progressively improving* the enjoyment of all people to the right to health and other health-related human rights. In working towards the goal of human rights and particularly the right to health, a rights-based approach upholds human rights standards and guiding principles, including but not limited to non-discrimination and equality, participation and inclusion, and accountability. (UN CESCR, 2000; UN CESCR, 2003).

Individual interventions

The individual approach focuses on high-risk or affected individuals through direct interventions. This can include interventions for primary prevention (e.g. a lifestyle intervention) in at-risk individuals. Secondary prevention strategies are aimed at decreasing mortality and the prevalence of ongoing or chronic complications in those who have been diagnosed with an illness. Population and individual approaches are complementary and function best when combined in an integrated manner (PAHO, 2011). Compare with **Population-based interventions**, see definition.

Intermediary determinants of health

Intermediary determinants are factors that shape people's health-related choices and outcomes and which are influenced by the **structural determinants** of health inequities. The main categories of intermediary determinants of health are:

- **Material circumstances:** Determinants linked to physical environments, including living conditions (e.g. housing and the neighbourhood, and working conditions) and consumption potential (e.g. funding to purchase healthy foods, clothing and other goods).

- **Psychosocial circumstances:** This includes psychosocial stressors, such as negative life events, stressful living conditions (e.g. high debt or financial insecurity) and lack of social support.

- **Behavioural and/or biological factors:** This includes smoking, diet, alcohol consumption and exercise. Depending on the pattern of exposure and vulnerability, behaviours may act as protective factors or to enhance health (e.g. exercise) or be harmful to health (e.g. cigarette smoking and obesity).

- **Health system:** The health system itself can directly intervene on differences in exposure and vulnerability, by ensuring equitable access to health services and the promotion of intersectoral action to improve health and well-being. The health system also acts as a mediating force or buffer against the impacts of an illness or disability on people's lives (Solar & Irwin, 2010).

See also **Mechanisms of social determinants**.

Intersectoral action

This refers to actions affecting health outcomes undertaken by sectors outside the health sector, possibly, but not necessarily, in collaboration with the health sector. Intersectoral action for health entails health and other sectors working together to inform public policy design and implementation to improve health and well-being, or, at least, not to adversely affect it. Such efforts improve understanding across health and other sectors about the way that the policy decisions and operational practices of different sectors impact on health and health equity (WHO, 2015b).

Inverse care law

The inverse care law refers to the availability of good medical care, which tends to vary inversely with the need for the population served. It operates more completely where medical care is most exposed to market forces, and less so where such exposure is reduced (Tudor Hart, 1971).

Key stages of the programme

The key stages of the programme include the organization of the programme and the sequences of interventions or activities that the programme undertakes to reach the potential changes or final results. The key stages are shown in a **programme diagram**.

Logic model

Logic model are activities illustrated graphically in a diagram that represents an overview of the programme, showing the sequences of activities with arrows connecting the relationships between them that combine to produce the changes that lead to the programme outcomes. Multiple logic models might be necessary to depict a broad, complex programme. In this case, a global model may illustrate the overall programme while more specific logic models depict different levels, components or stages within the global programme. These constitute "families of logic models" or "nested logic models" (Taylor-Powell & Henert, 2008).

Measures of social stratification

See **Socioeconomic position**.

Mechanisms of social determinants

- **Structural mechanisms** are those that generate stratification and social class divisions in society and that define individual socioeconomic position within hierarchies of power, prestige and access to resources. Structural mechanisms are rooted in the key institutions and processes of the socioeconomic and political context.

- **Intermediary mechanisms** are those through which intermediary determinants impact an individual's or group's health based on their relative socioeconomic positions, individuals and groups experience. Intermediary mechanisms include:

  - Different and unequal exposures to health;
  - Differential vulnerability as a result of these unequal exposures; and
  - Differential social, economic and health consequences as a result of these unequal exposures and vulnerabilities (Diderichsen et al, 2001).

Monitoring

Monitoring is a process that can help to determine the impact of policies, programmes and practices, and subsequently, to indicate whether change is needed. Generally speaking, monitoring is the process of repeatedly answering a given study question over time. In the world of policy, the study question usually pertains to the measurement of a condition that a policy seeks to impact. In this context, monitoring is useful and necessary as it has the ability to track policy outcomes over time and provides a means of evaluating the need for policy change. Once a policy has been changed, subsequent monitoring is necessary to evaluate the outcomes of the new policy, and thus monitoring should be an iterative and cyclical process that operates continuously (WHO, 2013c).

Population-based interventions

A population-based approach and interventions focus largely on health promotion activities and actions that influence the environment (i.e. physical, social, economic and regulatory). Population and individual approaches are complementary and function best when combined in an integrated manner (PAHO, 2011). Contrast with **Individual interventions**, see definition.

Problem space

Evidence for the problem space provides knowledge of what variables or systems of relationships are associated with health inequities (e.g. information on gradients of health inequities) (Sridharan, 2012). Contrast with **Solution space**, see definition.

Programme diagram

A programme diagram is a visual representation or model that shows the key stages of the programme to each of the intended changes or outcomes, and how these stages are organized and sequenced.

Programme goal, objectives and results

Programme goal is a broad statement describing the long-term ultimate aim of the programme. It serves as the foundation for developing programme objectives. Programme objectives describe the results to be achieved and how they will be achieved. Expected results are outcomes that a programme is designed to produce.

GLOSSARY OF KEY TERMS

Programme intervention

A programme intervention, service or activity refers to an action that enables attainment of one or more of the programme objectives, and hence serves to deliver the expected results. See **Individual interventions** and **Population-based interventions**.

Programme theory

See **Theory of the programme**.

Quality

Quality is one of the four elements of the right to health. It calls for health facilities, goods and services to be scientifically and medically appropriate and of good quality (CESCR, 2000). This requires skilled medical personnel; scientifically approved and unexpired drugs and hospital equipment; safe and potable water; and adequate sanitation, among other inputs. Issues such as a strong referral network, as well as attention to issues such as treatment adherence, diagnostic accuracy, and provider compliance, are important for quality in the context of effective coverage (UN CESCR, 2000).

Realist evaluation

Realist evaluation places emphasis on: (i) identifying the mechanisms that produce observable effects of the programme; and (ii) testing these mechanisms and other context variables that may have impacts on the observed effects. The focus is on developing explanations of the consequences of social actions that contribute to the greater understanding of *why, where and for whom health programmes work or fail*. It also recognizes the complexity of the transformation processes sought by programmes, and the importance of context and influence of policies and programmes from other sectors (Pawson & Tilley, 2004).

See also **Theory-driven evaluation**.

Results chain of programme

- **Inputs:** Resources that go into the programme and how they are organized for service delivery, including: staff (type), facilities, money, materials, equipment and volunteer time (i.e. what is invested).

- **Outputs:** The goods, services or other activities delivered by the programme. The programme outputs are often described in terms of quantitative productivity (i.e. what the programme does and who it reaches). Outputs are different from outcomes. While outcomes describe the actual impact (the change that results), outputs simply describe the quantity of services provided (Taylor-Powell & Henert, 2008).

- **Outcomes and impacts:** The results or changes from the programme that may be expressed in a continuum: usually target population service coverage indicators are associated with outcomes. Outcomes can be immediate or short term, intermediate, final or long term. Impact typically refers to changes in morbidity and mortality that have been influenced (acknowledging issues of attribution) by the coverage rates of the population with a set of services (i.e. what results the programme is expected to achieve).

Right to health

The WHO Constitution was the first international instrument to enshrine the enjoyment of the highest attainable standard of health as a fundamental right of every human being ("the right to health"). It has since been recognized in numerous international law instruments, including the International Covenant on Economic, Social and Cultural Rights (1966). The right to health in international human rights law is a claim to a set of social arrangements – norms, institutions, laws and an enabling environment – that can best secure the enjoyment of this right. It is an inclusive right extending not only to timely and appropriate health care but also to the underlying determinants of health, for example access to health information, access to water and food, housing, etc.

The right to health is subject to progressive realization and acknowledges resource constraints. However, it also imposes on states various obligations which are of immediate effect, such as the guarantee that the right will be exercised without discrimination of any kind and the obligation to take deliberate, concrete and targeted steps towards its full realization (WHO, 2015c). The right to health draws attention to four interrelated and essential elements, namely availability, accessibility, acceptability and quality (CESCR, 2000).

Social capital

While there is no single definition of social capital, the key feature is that social capital refers to an intangible, dynamic and collective resource for societies that facilitates social relationships and connections. It includes elements such as trust, participation, social support and reciprocity. A high level of social capital and social cohesion works to protect people's health and well-being, including by addressing discrimination, marginalization and exclusion. Inequality can contribute to a breakdown in social cohesion and social capital.

Social class

Social class is defined by relations of ownership or control over productive resources (i.e. physical, financial and organizational). Social class provides an explicit relational mechanism (property, management) that explains how economic inequalities are generated and how they may affect health. The WHO conceptual framework of the social determinants of health positions social class as one component of **socioeconomic position** (Solar & Irwin, 2010).

Social determinants of health

The social determinants of health are the conditions in which people are born, grow, live, work and age, including the health system. These circumstances are shaped by the distribution of money, power and resources at global, national and local levels, which are themselves influenced by policy choices (WHO, 2015d). See also **Intermediary determinants of health** and **Structural determinants**.

Social gradient

The term social gradient in health refers to the stepwise or linear decrease in health that comes with decreasing social position (Marmot, 2004). The impact of the social gradient is sometimes expressed as a shortfall in health, that is, the number of lives that would have been saved if all groups in society had the same high level of health as the most advantaged group (Whitehead & Dahlgren, 2006).

Social groups

Structural societal factors determine a social hierarchy in which different groups have unequal positions. Social groups can be defined by gender, ethnicity, sexuality, social class, socioeconomic position (income, occupation), territory, disability and/or age. Since the social position of the group defines the access to the social resources, as opportunities for health, and their exposure to risks associated with health lasts throughout the vital cycle, even between generations (Krieger, 2002). The participants must identify the most relevant social groups for equity analysis.

Social participation

Social participation concerns the participation of civil society and the empowerment of affected communities to become active protagonists in shaping their own health. All persons and groups are entitled to active, free and meaningful participation in, contribution to, and enjoyment of civil, economic, social, cultural and political development in which human rights and fundamental freedoms can be realized (UNDG, 2003). Human rights law recognizes the participation of the population in all health-related decision-making at the community, national and international levels (CESCR, 2000). Participation is one of the human rights principles that needs to be considered when applying a human rights-based approach to health. Adequate and sustainable financial and technical support, including investment in empowerment of rights-holders, is essential to enable meaningful participation.

Similarly, social determinants of health frameworks draw attention to social participation. It is the role, power and control of social groups in decisions and actions that shape their own health. In relation to programmes, participation may take different forms: information, advisory, deliberative or empowerment. It can also be distinguished if participation is motivated by claims of self interests, whether by individual or by collective issues at the social justice scope. That is, if participation contributes to the redistribution of power or not (Solar & Irwin, 2010).

Socioeconomic position

Socioeconomic position refers to the social and economic factors that influence the position that individuals or groups hold within the structure of a society. It is a term that encompasses the various measures, referring to the position of individuals or groups in the social hierarchy. It is understood

GLOSSARY OF KEY TERMS

as an aggregate concept that includes integrated measurement of access to resources and prestige in society, linking these with social class (Marx, Weber, Krieger, Williams and Moss) (Solar & Irwin, 2010) coupled with growing inequalities in income and wealth, have refocused attention on social class as a key determinant of population health. Routine analysis using conceptually coherent and consistent measures of socioeconomic position in US public health research and surveillance, however, remains rare. This review discusses concepts and methodologies concerning, and guidelines for measuring, social class and other aspects of socioeconomic position (e.g. income, poverty, deprivation, wealth, education. A variety of other terms, such as social class, social stratum and social or socioeconomic status, are often used more or less interchangeably in the literature, despite their different theoretical bases.

Socioeconomic position is an integrated concept about social stratification processes that considers three key components:

• **Resource-based processes:** Refer to material and social resources and assets, including income, wealth, and educational credentials; terms used to describe inadequate resources include "poverty" and "deprivation".

• **Prestige-based processes:** Refer to an individual ranking or status in the social hierarchy, typically evaluated in terms of the level in magnitude and quality of access and consumption of goods, services and knowledge. These measures include occupation, education and income, which relate to prestige in given contexts. This is linked to the concept of **social class** (Solar & Irwin, 2010).

• **Discrimination-based processes:** For example, "gender" refers to those characteristics of women and men which are socially constructed, whereas "sex" designates those characteristics that are biologically determined. Gender involves "culture-bound conventions, roles and behaviours" that shape relations between and among women and men and boys and girls (Borrell et al, 2014; WHO, 2011). In many societies, gender constitutes a fundamental basis for discrimination, which can be defined as the process by which members of a socially defined group are treated differently, especially unfairly because of their inclusion in that group.

Solution space

The solution space offers knowledge of what kinds of interventions are likely to work, for whom and under what contexts (Sridharan, 2012). Contrast with the **Problem space**, see definition.

Stratification

The term stratification is used in sociology to refer to social hierarchies in which individuals or groups can be arranged along a ranked order of some attribute, such as income or years of education. Measures of social stratification (using equity stratifiers) are important predictors of patterns of mortality and morbidity, and are therefore used to monitor health inequality. This information is important to assess and inform policies, programmes and practices in order to reduce differences in health that are unfair and unjust. Some of the most frequently used stratifiers are: income or wealth; place of residence (rural, urban, other); race or ethnicity; occupation (workers/ employed, unemployed); sex; religion; education; socioeconomic status; social class; age; and gender identity and sexual orientation.

Structural determinants

Structural determinants are the underlying social determinants of health inequities and include socioeconomic and political context, structural mechanisms that generate stratification and social class divisions, and the resultant socioeconomic position of individuals. The socioeconomic and political context includes aspects such as the labour market, the educational system, political institutions and redistributive policies as well as cultural and societal values (Solar & Irwin, 2010).

See also **Mechanisms of social determinants**.

Tanahashi model of effective coverage

The Tanahashi model of effective programme coverage examines five domains of health service delivery performance. These domains are **Availability, Accessibility, Acceptability, Contact coverage** and **Effective coverage,** which can be drawn as a coverage curve. The model aims to support evaluation to identify bottlenecks in the operation of the service, to analyse the constraining factors responsible for such bottlenecks, and to select effective measures for service development (Tanahashi, 1978). The Tanahashi domains are similar but not to be confused with the four interrelated elements of the right to health, namely availability, accessibility, acceptability and quality.

Target population

Refers to the population that is eligible to use or the beneficiary of either a health service or social guarantees of other sectors. It is the population for whom the service or the guarantee is intended.

Theory-driven evaluation

Theory-driven evaluation (or programme theory-driven evaluation) is a contextual or holistic assessment of a programme based on the conceptual framework of programme theory (see **Theory of a programme**). The purpose of theory-driven evaluation is to provide information on not only the performance or merit of a programme but on how and why the programme achieves such a result. It provides insightful information that assists stakeholders in understanding those components of their programme that work well and those that do not (Pawson & Tilley, 2004; Chen, 1990). See also **Realist evaluation**.

Theory of inequities

A theory of inequities explains why inequities occur in relation to programme access and benefits. It helps identifying the key entry points and opportunities for adjusting the programme to better address the coverage and equity gaps.

Theory of the programme

The theory of a programme can be described as the representation of the mechanisms by which means it is understood that the programme activities contribute to the expected outcomes, in the short, medium and long term. It is a model that specifies what must be done to achieve the objectives, and to understand what actually happens in each key stage of the programme (Rogers, 2008).

Types of coverage

See **Universal, mixed, selective/targeted coverage**.

Universal health coverage

The goal of universal health coverage is to ensure that all people obtain the health services they need without suffering financial hardship when paying for them (WHO, 2015e). The services must be of adequate quality and cover the whole continuum of care (promotion, prevention, treatment, rehabilitation and palliation). Universal health coverage is firmly based on the WHO Constitution of 1948 declaring health a fundamental human right and on the Health for All agenda set by the Alma-Ata Declaration in 1978. Equity is paramount. Universal health coverage is a means through which to operationalize commitments to equity and the right to health.

Universal, selective/targeted, mixed coverage

- **Universal coverage:** When considering programmes, universal coverage means intervention coverage or access is provided to the whole population of a country who has a specific health need, usually under the principle of citizenship benefits or rights. These interventions are designed to benefit all people with that health need, regardless of their personal, social and economic characteristics (Raczynski, 1995).

- **Selective/"targeted" coverage:** The intervention coverage or access is allocated on a selective basis, usually determined by an assessment of need (for example, as determined by means testing of income).

- **Mixed coverage:** The intervention coverage or access is a combination of universal and selective coverage, where the selectivity is used as an instrument to enforce or strengthen universalism. This has been referred to as "targeting within universalism", whereby the additional benefits are targeted to priority or high-need subpopulations (e.g. the lowest income group) in the context of a universal policy (Mkandawire, 2005).

GLOSSARY OF KEY TERMS

REFERENCES

Borrell C, Palència L, Muntaner C, Urquía M, Malmusi D, O'Campo P (2014). Influence of macrosocial policies on women's health and gender inequalities in health. Epidemiologic Reviews. 2014;36(1):31–48. Available: http://epirev.oxfordjournals.org/content/36/1/31.abstract (accessed 24 February 2016).

Chen HT (1990). Theory-Driven Evaluations. Sage.

Diderichsen F, Evans T, Whitehead M (2001). The social basis of disparities in health. In: Evans T et al, eds. Challenging inequities in health. New York: Oxford University Press.

Krieger N (2002). A glossary for social epidemiology. Epidemiological Bulletin. 2002;23(1):7–11.

Marmot M (2004). The status syndrome: how social standing affects our health and longevity. London: Bloomsbury Publishing. Available: http://www.amazon.co.uk/Status-Syndrome-Standing - Affects Longevity/dp/0805073701 (accessed 4 March 2016).

Ministerio de Salud, Chile (2010). Documento Técnico III. Guía para analizar equidad en el acceso y los resultados de los programas y su relación con los DSS. Santiago: Subsecretaria de Salud Pública. Ministry of Health, Chile (2010). Technical document III. Guide for the equity analysis on programmes' access and results and their link with social determinants of health. Santiago: Undersecretary for Public Health.] Materials in Spanish only. Available: http://www.superacionpobreza.cl/wp-content/uploads/2014/03/guia_para_analizar.pdf (accessed 4 March 2016).

Ministry of Health, Social Services and Equality, Government of Spain (2012). Methodological guide to integrate equity into health strategies, programmes and activities. Version 1. Madrid. Available: http://www.msssi.gob.es/profesionales/saludPublica/prevPromocion/promocion/desigualdadSalud/jornadaPresent_Guia2012/docs/Methodological_Guide_Equity_SPAs.pdf (accessed 17 February 2016).

Mkandawire T (2005). Targeting and Universalism in Poverty Reduction. United Nations Research Institute for Social Development. Social Policy and Development Programme Paper Number 23. Geneva: UNRISD. Available: http://www.unrisd.org/80256B3C005BCCF9/search/955FB8A594EEA0B0C12570FF00493EAA?OpenDocument (accessed 18 February 2016).

Narayan D (2005). Measuring empowerment: Cross-disciplinary perspectives. Washington, DC: The World Bank. Available: https://openknowledge.worldbank.org/bitstream/handle/10986/7441/344100PAPER0Me101Official0use0only1.pdf?sequence=1 (accessed 25 February 2016).

OHCHR (2014). What are human rights? Geneva: Office of the High Commissioner for Human Rights. Available: http://www.ohchr.org/EN/Issues/Pages/WhatareHumanRights.aspx (accessed 4 March 2016).

PAHO (Pan American Health Organization) (2011). Population and individual approaches to the prevention and management of diabetes and obesity. Washington, DC: PAHO. Available: http://www.paho.org/hq./index.php?option=com_docman&task=doc_view&gid=15557&Itemid (accessed 4 March 2016).

Pawson R, Sridharan S (2009). Theory-driven evaluation of public health programmes. In: Killoran A, Kelly M, eds. Evidence-based public health: Effectiveness and efficiency. Oxford: Oxford University Press: 43–61.

Pawson R, Tilley N (2004). Realist Evaluation. London: British Cabinet Office. Available: http://www.communitymatters.com.au/RE_chapter.pdf (accessed 18 February 2016).

Raczynski D (1995). "Introduction" and "Programs, Institutions, and Resources: Chile". In: Raczynski D, ed. Strategies to Combat Poverty in Latin America. Washington, DC: Inter-American Development Bank.

Rogers PJ (2008). Using programme theory to evaluate complicated and complex aspects of interventions. Evaluation. 2008;14(1):29–48. Available: http://evi.sagepub.com/content/14/1/29.full.pdf+html (accessed 4 March 2016).

Solar O, Irwin A (2010). A conceptual framework for action on the social determinants of health. Social Determinants of Health Discussion Paper 2 (Policy and Practice). Geneva: World Health Organization. Available: http://www.who.int/sdhconference/resources/ConceptualframeworkforactiononSDH_eng.pdf (accessed 26 February 2016).

Sridharan S (2012). A Pocket Guide to Evaluating Health Equity Interventions – Some Questions for Reflection by Sanjeev Sridharan. Magic: Measuring & Managing Access Gaps in Care (blog entry). Available: http://www.longwoods.com/blog/a-pocket-guide-to-evaluating-health-equity-interventions-some-questions-for-reflection/, (accessed 17 February 2016).

Tanahashi T (1978). Health service coverage and its evaluation. Bulletin of the World Health Organization. 1978;56(2):295–303.

Taylor-Powell E, Henert E (2008). Developing a logic model: Teaching and training guide. Madison, WI: University of Wisconsin-Extension Cooperative Extension, Program Development and Evaluation. Available: http://www.uwex.edu/ces/pdande/evaluation/evallogicmodel.html (accessed 18 February 2016).

Tudor Hart J (1971). The Inverse Care Law. Lancet. 1971;297(7696):405–12. Available: http://www.thelancet.com/article/S014067367192410X/fulltext (accessed 4 March 2016).

UN CESCR (Committee on Economic, Social and Cultural Rights) (2000). General Comment No. 14: The Right to the Highest Attainable Standard of Health (Art. 12 of the Covenant), 11 August 2000, E/C.12/2000/4. Available: http://www.refworld.org/docid/4538838d0.html (accessed 4 March 2016).

UN CESCR (Committee on Economic, Social and Cultural Rights) (2003). General Comment No. 15: The Right to Water (Arts. 11 and 12 of the Covenant), 20 January 2003, E/C.12/2002/11. Available from: http://www.refworld.org/docid/4538838d11.html (accessed 4 March 2016).

UN CESCR (Committee on Economic, Social and Cultural Rights) (2009). General Comment No. 20: Non-Discrimination in Economic, Social and Cultural Rights, 02 July 2009, E/C.12/GC/20. Available: http://www.refworld.org/docid/4a60961f2.html (accessed 8 March 2016).

UN HRBA Portal (2016). The Human Rights Based Approach to Development Cooperation: Towards a Common Understanding Among UN Agencies. Available: http://hrbaportal.org/the-human-rights-based-approach-to-development-cooperation-towards-a-common-understanding-among-un-agencies#sthash.wN2ZbC4G.dpuf (accessed 2 March 2016).

UNDG (2003). The Human Rights Based Approach to Development Cooperation Towards a Common Understanding Among UN Agencies. New York, United Nations Development Group. Available: https://undg.org/main/undg_document/the-human-rights-based-approach-to-development-cooperation-towards-a-common-understanding-among-un-agencies/ (accessed 5 March 2016).

UNEG (2012). Norms for Evaluation in the UN System. New York: United Nations Evaluation Group. Available: http://www.uneval.org/document/detail/21 (accessed 5 March 2016).

Whitehead M, Dahlgren G (2006). Levelling up (part 1): a discussion paper on on concepts and principles for tackling social inequities in health. Copenhagen: WHO Regional Office for Europe.

WHO (2010). Equity, social determinants and public health programmes. Geneva: World Health Organization. Available: http://whqlibdoc.who.int/publications/2010/9789241563970_eng.pdf (accessed 22 February 2016).

WHO (2011). Gender mainstreaming for health managers: a practical approach. Geneva: World Health Organization. Available: http://www.who.int/gender/documents/health_managers_guide/en/ (access 24 February 2016).

WHO (2013a). Women's and children's health: Evidence of impact of human rights. Bustreo F, Hunt P, eds. Geneva: World Health Organization. Available: http://apps.who.int/iris/bitstream/10665/84203/1/9789241505420_eng.pdf?ua=1 (accessed 4 March 2016).

WHO (2013b). WHO Evaluation Practice Handbook. Geneva: World Health Organization. Available: http://apps.who.int/iris/bitstream/10665/96311/1/9789241548687_eng.pdf (accessed 27 February 2016).

WHO (2013c). Handbook on health inequality monitoring – with a special focus on low- and middle-income countries. Geneva: World Health Organization. Available: http://apps.who.int/iris/bitstream/10665/85345/1/9789241548632_eng.pdf?ua=1 (accessed 24 February 2016).

WHO (2014a). Ensuring human rights in the provision of contraceptive information and services: Guidance and recommendations. Geneva: World Health Organization. Available: http://apps.who.int/iris/bitstream/10665/102539/1/9789241506748_eng.pdf?ua=1 (accessed 4 March 2016).

WHO (WHA67.12) (2014b). Contributing to social and economic development: sustainable action across sectors to improve health and health equity. Geneva, Sixty-Seventh World Health Assembly. Available: http://apps.who.int/gb/ebwha/pdf_files/WHA67/A67_R12-en.pdf (accessed 4 March 2016).

WHO (2015a). Glossary of terms used. Health impact assessment. World Health Organization. Available: http://www.who.int/hia/about/glos/en/ (accessed 8 March 2016).

WHO (2015b). Health in All Policies Training Manual. Geneva: World Health Organization. Available: http://apps.who.int/iris/bitstream/10665/151788/1/9789241507981_eng.pdf (accessed 2 March 2016).

WHO (2015c). Health and Human Rights. Geneva: World Health Organization. Available: http://www.who.int/mediacentre/factsheets/fs323/en/index.html (accessed 4 March 2016).

WHO (2015d). Social determinants of health. Geneva: World Health Organization. Available: http://www.who.int/social_determinants/en/ (accessed 4 March 2016).

WHO (2015e). What is universal health coverage? Geneva: World Health Organization. Available: http://www.who.int/features/qa/universal_health_coverage/en/index.html (accessed 4 March 2016).

WHO and Ministry of Social Affairs and Health, Government of Finland (2013). Helsinki Statement on Health in All Policies 2013. Statement of the 8th Global Conference on Health Promotion, Helsinki, Finland, 10–14 June 2013. Available: http://www.who.int/healthpromotion/conferences/8gchp/8gchp_helsinki_statement.pdf (accessed 4 March 2016).

WHO and OHCHR (2015). A human rights-based approach to health. Information sheet. Available: http://www.ohchr.org/Documents/Issues/ESCR/Health/HRBA_HealthInformationSheet.pdf (accessed 4 March 2016).

WHO Regional Office for Europe (2008). The Tallinn Charter: Health Systems for Health and Wealth. Copenhagen. Available: http://www.euro.who.int/__data/assets/pdf_file/0008/88613/E91438.pdf (accessed 4 March 2016).